The
SECRET
ART
of
HEALTH
&
FITNESS

The

SECRET

ART

of

HEALTH

&

FITNESS

Uncovered from
the Martial Arts Masters

Claudio A. Iedwab *&* Roxanne L. Standefer

WEATHERHILL
New York • Tokyo

$3/_{00}$

First edition, 1999

© 1999 Claudio A. Iedwab & Roxanne L. Standefer
Artwork & Illustrations © 1999 Claudio A. Iedwab
Cover Photograph © 1999 Roxanne L. Standefer

99   00   01   02   03   04   5   4   3   2   1

Library of Congress Cataloging-in-Publication Data
Iedwab, Claudio A.
The secret art of health and fitness: uncovered from the martial arts masters / Claudio A. Iedwab, Roxanne L. Standefer.
p. cm.   x, 163 p.   Bib. p. 161-163
Includes bibliographical references and index.
ISBN 0-8348-0462-X
1. Martial arts--Health aspects. 2. Exercise--Health aspects.
I. Standefer, Roxanne L. II. Title.
RA781.I33 1999
613.7'148--dc21
                                                    99-27000
                                                    CIP

To all the *sensei*, both present and gone before,
especially Sensei Uensei, who taught us the simplicity of:
breathe, relax, and smile . . .

Contents

Preface

THIS book is about the martial arts from our point of view. We hope that we have made it clear that there are as many ways to walk this path as there are other paths to follow, both old and new. We have tried to distill and synthesize the basic principles of the many martial arts, and explain the reasons for their disparate development and their legacy as the original mind-body exercise system. Although myths are exploded and secrets revealed, every effort has been made to respect the original intentions of the founders of the modern martial arts and the masters of the ancient traditions.

The Secret Art of Health & Fitness is intended for martial artists of all styles, but also for anyone interested in physical education, body movement, health and healing, and certainly Asian culture and philosophy. We welcome comments and dialogue about the issues raised. Readers of this book will not necessarily find that all schools of martial art share our analysis or practices, but many do. We hope that, as more people become familiar with the rich tradition of holistic improvement embodied in the training, those who deny the "art" in martial art and aspire to no philosophy behind their punch, kick, or throw, will leave the field and go fight amongst themselves.

Our own path is *Gorindo*, "the Friendly Martial Art," founded in Canada by Claudio in 1990. As both teachers and students of this non-competitive school, we strongly advocate the role of martial arts in the development of the health and fitness, both mental and physical, of all individuals. We believe in a spirituality that is connected with nature, and teach that everyone has to come to terms with his or her own place in the universe. It is not for us to say what that may be.

Nevertheless, writing a book about such a complex subject meant that we had to make choices, express some opinions, and generally simplify ideas and information. The more we explained, the more we felt needed to be said, to the point where every chapter could become another book. Trusting in the Zen adage that "less is more," and relying on our own experiences and research in the martial arts, will certainly result in errors and omissions, which are our responsibility entirely. Similarly, we had to grapple with making generalizations about Eastern and Western culture, traditions, and teachings, not always appropriate in a world of global communication and infinite diversity; yet in some cases it was necessary to briefly explain traditional differences. We also had to deal with the problem of the lack of a neutral pronoun in the English language. After some deliberation, and entertaining the idea of she being the teacher (as females often are in the natural world) and he being everyone else, we decided to follow the convention of using he throughout, when we could not form the sentence otherwise. We felt comfortable that in the martial arts "she" has always included "he" and that it was the intention of the founders that the teachings were for everyone on an equal basis. Certainly this gender neutrality is true in *gorindo*, whereof we are most qualified to speak.

We are extremely grateful to our publisher, Weatherhill, for including us in their *dojo* as white belts, and to Ray Furse, editorial director, for his enthusiasm for the book and his quiet, incisive way with us. We are indebted to our students, assistant instructors and stewards for their support, patience, and extraordinary willingness to learn, and our friends and family for their encouragement. And finally, to each other for helping to bring out the best. With *kiai*, for all of you!

Claudio & Roxanne

The

SECRET
ART
of
HEALTH
&
FITNESS

Chapter 1

Why the Big Secret?

MARTIAL artists have always sought high levels of fitness. From the early Shaolin monks, who trained to improve their health, to the movie stars of the moment who want to look good for their fans, there have been a variety of reasons and methods for attaining a strong, healthy body. What sets the martial arts apart from most other exercise systems is their stress on the integration of the mind with the body. Emphasis on integrity, excellence, and harmony of spirit is fundamental to all traditions. Furthermore, what makes a martial art unique is the philosophy of learning through which it is approached.

It is a testament to the strength of these traditions that martial arts in a very pure sense can still be practiced in the modern world, and in some rare cases, remain relatively untouched by the passage of time. Where this is not the case, the reasons are many. While nearly everyone is aware of the existance of the martial arts, not everyone knows what they are really about. In the modern era they continue to suffer from a dual perception, on the one hand regarded as the epitome of serious athletic skill and mastery, and on the other, ridiculed as a sport in which guys in pyjamas jump around and shriek like banshees. Every martial artist has had the experience of discussing their practice with someone who jokingly shies away and blurts out an inane comment like: "I better not be getting in *your* way" or "I hope you won't *hurt* me." However, while some might think martial arts are too violent, most people respect the need for self-defense skills, although fewer are aware of the deeper philosophies that underlie the study of martial arts.

The human body has not changed much in the past thousand years and certainly not in the past hundred. Evolution has not shielded the

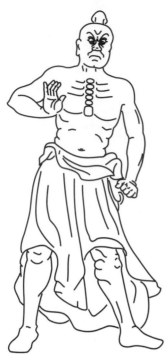

Statues of guardian warriors were erected for protection even at sacred precincts such as temples and shrines.

vulnerable and sensitive organism that is *homo sapiens* from the many ravages of its environment. We still puncture easily, succumb to cold and heat, and if the holes on the front of the head are covered for more than a few minutes, we suffocate and die. Compared to other earthly creatures we haven't developed much in the way of hard shells, sharp teeth, or fast legs to help us in our self-defense. Nevertheless, our species keeps stumbling along, aided by our success at propagation and our reliance upon our supposedly advanced mental capacities to survive. Proponents of human supremacy in the course of evolution note that only man is capable of art, invention, and philosophy. Our brains have substituted construction, clothing, and weapons (technology) for natural protection. It might be argued that our excellence at wielding such "tools" may prove to be the downfall of the human race. No other organism on the planet has the propensity to pollute its nest and exterminate its kind, to the extent that its own survival and that of the entire ecosystem is threatened. Given such possibilities, how great, really, is our capacity for self-defense?

Survival and defense techniques and methods for transmitting this knowledge have existed since the beginning of mankind. Animal and plant species have this knowledge as well, although we tend to refer to instinct or survival mechanisms when speaking of non-human social organization. In human societies based on a hunter-gatherer culture, techniques of killing for food and means of protecting territories from invaders have been passed down through the generations in a variety of ways. Many of our traditional art forms, including painting, dancing, and storytelling have evolved from this transmission.

The role of the warrior in society was honored out of necessity, and usually involved respect for a strict code of behavior, discipline, and special knowledge. Even the most peaceful societies have recognized the need for the defense of their way of life from those who would disrupt it. It seems an unfortunate reality of the human condition that the potential for violent conflict exists. History has shown that man can always find some reason to fight, and devotes much of his resources to that end. To some theorists, the advancement of civilization, in terms of technology, social organization, and discovery, has depended on it. Yet, in our utopian visions, it is a truly advanced society that can turn its energies towards beauty and advancement of knowledge that improves the human condition.

The history of modern martial arts has roots primarily in Eastern Asia, although its influences and effects can be considered global. Some of these traditions have evolved from those of the samurai of feudal Japan but the modern martial arts of *karate-do, taekwondo, judo,* and others, are twentieth century disciplines. The study of martial arts as a way of life for improving health, spirit, and character goes back much farther, to a different time and place.

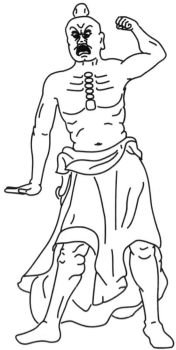

Most histories of the martial arts point to the arrival in central China in 520 A.D. of a Buddhist monk from India as a significant event in their development. It is said that Bodhidharma took up residence at the Shaolin temple and taught the monks techniques for breathing and meditation, along with exercises for health and self-defense. They were interested in this knowledge as a way to keep them healthy during long periods of study and devotion. They also needed to protect them-

The warrior spirit of temple guardians was believed able to sway the intentions of those who intended harm.

selves from waves of violent political oppression and from highway robbers, who would attack them as they traveled through the country alone. Their priestly vows prevented them from using weapons.

Bodhidharma established a Buddhist sect called Chan that later spread to Japan, where it was called Zen, the name by which it is more widely known today. The previously established Confucian and Taoist ideals of early Chinese thinkers (circa 600 B.C.), also became mixed with Chan philosophy and religion as it moved throughout China and neighboring regions. Itinerant monks, envoys, and merchants carried this knowledge to the island of Okinawa and the Ryukyu island chain from where it eventually spread to Japan. Korea also received such waves of visitation and some of the principles were incorporated into the teaching of its fighting techniques.

Respect for elders and the relationship of a student to a *sensei* (literally, "one who has gone before") is an important concept that influenced the transmission of martial arts knowledge. Another fundamental concept is that of the *tao* (in Chinese; *do* in Japanese), loosely defined as the Way, a philosophical approach that emphasizes self-improvement. This philosophy teaches that more important than acquiring technique, was the process of traveling the path of learning. The goal was education of the ego and acquiring an understanding of how the mind worked.

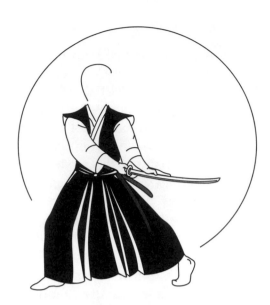

*The Way of the samurai included
an obligation to defend their
feudal masters.*

The incorporation of this ideal is thought to be a major difference between the development of Eastern and Western ways of thinking and artistic expression.

Combat techniques, as a body of knowledge, became known in Japan as *bujutsu* and the fighter as a *bushi*. The warrior classes had varying degrees of political clout throughout Japanese history. Although sometimes holding absolute power, they were just as often consigned to the servitude of a particular master. The samurai were an example of a class of warrior who were thus bound; their code of honor, conduct, and the commitment to die for their masters, similar to the code of chivalry for European knights, was known as *bushido*.

Those unfamiliar with details of Japanese history have painted the samurai as mythic figures who ranged widely about the land and through all the centuries, yet the periods to which the legends refer and those which inform the martial arts of today, are much more specific. Despite their rigid codes of behavior, there were both good and bad samurai. In trying to understand the influence of martial history on modern schools, one must distinguish between the training and accomplishments of armies for organized warfare, and the more individual preparations, attitudes, and achievements of the classical warrior.

Another major development occurred in Japan between the fourteenth and seventeenth centuries. Warrior clans of the samurai class began to organize their fighting skills into *ryu*, or schools, in order to transmit the most effective techniques along family or household lines. These thousands of schools varied according to strategy, weapons used, and the geographical realities in the areas of those who created them. Fighting in the mountains was different from fighting on sandy beaches, for example. These *ryu* held their methods very secretively, and loyalty to the founders and current heads of the school was paramount.

In general, a true *ryu* was founded based on mystical experience or attainment of Zen enlightenment, *satori*, on the part of the founder, who then felt compelled to study and build upon the principles illuminated. Where traditions and techniques were eventually recorded in sacred scrolls, the information was often in a cryptic code and guarded quite closely. Even today, descendants of these traditional schools are careful about how and with whom this information is shared.

After 1603 Japan entered a more peaceful era known as the Edo period. The establishment of the Tokugawa Shogunate ended much of the feudal warfare of the past and created at least the facade of a stable society, based on rigid social classes and isolation from the outside world. There was less demand for the samurai warrior with unswerving loyalty to his master, and as a result the diverse fighting *ryu* began to develop more into arts. As the many weapons of warfare fell into disuse there was more interest in the training of unarmed techniques of fighting, known as *jujutsu*. As well, in the more cultured society the samurai was obliged to learn other arts beside those of the warrior. Calligraphy, poetry, painting, gardening, and the game of *go*, were all part of his daily life. He honed his intellect and creativity as keenly as his sword. He practiced these arts to focus his mind and calm himself before battle, but more importantly to remind himself of what was good in life and worth fighting for. The exquisite formalities of the tea ceremony were much revered and practiced as a display of self-control, grace, and simple beauty. This change in Japanese society and the influence of the Zen and Taoist teachings led to the study of martial arts as a "way" of life, and they became known as *budo*.

Bu is translated as "martial," or "warlike," but a different meaning is conveyed when the word is written in *kanji*, the ideographic pictograms for writing borrowed by the Japanese from the Chinese. The original symbol for war, representing the spear or sword, is joined by other lines indicating the *stopping* of the spear to end the conflict. It is this defensive and peaceful intention that is often lost in the translation of

Bu: *stop conflict*

bu in Western languages. The *do* suffix further expands the concept from things warlike by emphasizing creativity and concentration of energy on a path of learning.

Many other Japanese and Korean arts use the word *do* to identify them as lifelong studies guided by a master. *Karate-do, judo, aikido, kendo, kyudo, iaido, taekwondo,* etc., of the martial line and also the arts of flower arranging, calligraphy, the tea ceremony, and even the strategic game of *go*, are all *do*. These arts are further connected to martial traditions by having *dan* grading levels and rules for the transmission of teachings from master to student within *ryu* or school lines.

JIGORO KANO (1860–1938) studied and adapted the traditional hand-to-hand combat techniques of *jujutsu* and formed a school known as *kodokan judo* (the gentle way) in 1882. He used basic principles of physics and body mechanics to design a training method that minimized injury. Concentration and focus of energy to maximize the efficiency of technique was paramount, with the principle of "giving way" to eventually overcome being fundamental to the art. Later, *judo* followed the sporting path into the Olympic Games.

GICHIN FUNAKOSHI (1868–1957) is considered the father of modern *karate-do* (the way of the empty hand) because he introduced Okinawan *naha-te* and *shuri-te* traditions to Japan in 1916 and 1922. Forming a friendship with Jigoro Kano, he decided to remain and live in Japan, where he established his own school that later became known as *shotokan* style, one of the most widely practiced *ryu* of *karate-do* today. Funakoshi devoted much of his time to writing and traveling, teaching both technique and a philosophical basis for martial art. He did not believe in competition and began the teaching of *karate-do* in schools for young people.

MORIHEI UESHIBA (1883–1969) influenced a different line with his school of *aiki budo* (1925) which became known as *aikido* (the way of harmony of energy) around 1941, referred to later in his writings as the "art of peace." His emphasis on the spiritual aspect of the martial arts and the non-competition, non-confrontational approach to the teaching has had a significant influence.

There are numerous fighting disciplines and martial art styles from countries and cultures that are very old and which may have had roots in India or China. *Kalaripayit, shorinji kempo, pakua, hsing-i chuan, pentjak silat, tae-kyon, muay thai, bando,* and *kushti* are just a few examples. Some have developed in a completely different manner due to unusual circumstances, such as *capoeira* (a Brazilian kicking and dance movement with its roots in the slave trade from Africa). *Savate,* French boxing, is another independent example.

While almost all nations and cultures have warrior or military traditions, and many have seen their historical practices manifested in dance and sports, historically, it has been in Asia where martial arts, as a way of life embodying physical, mental, and spiritual practice, have flourished. The exchange of technique and ideas through visits of travelers and the wanderings of itinerant monks has somehow managed to mix many influences that have given a common weight and history to the martial arts, while they individually continue to grow and diversify.

Political upheavals and cultural changes have influenced the evolution of martial arts. Invasions of one country by another have created underground fighting styles in reaction to such oppression. For example, when the Japanese invaded and occupied the island of Okinawa they banned all weapons. The local farmers and fishermen adapted their tools as weapons, which have become the *kama, tonfa, eku, bo,* and *nunchaku* practiced today as the traditional weapons. Many martial arts incorporated elements of dance or theater in order to camouflage training in them during times of oppression. In China, traditional lines of *kung fu* (defined as "an art one excels in") and *wushu* (the gymnastic, dance-like martial forms) with its own variation in styles, techniques, and masters continues into modern times. *Tai chi chuan* as well has had a tremendous growth in Western society as its relationship to health, breathing and *chi* energy (*ki* in Japanese) has become recognized. Korea had its own class of ancient military knights known as the *hwa rang*. But it was the influence of Chinese fighting techniques and the occupation of Korea by Japan from 1910 through 1945 that are thought more likely to have affected the development of the modern schools of Korean martial art such as *taekwondo*.

Most of the popularly recognized martial arts, such as *karate-do, judo, aikido*, and *taekwondo*, have been formulated only in the last hundred years. The founders of these martial arts, and the teachers who followed them, managed to establish these lines strongly in the existing firmament of styles. Despite offshoots and distortions due to modern commercialism and competition, the ideals that they promoted and their stature as historic figures are undiminished, primarily because of the depth of the teachings and the writings they left behind. However, all these schools have numerous variations, style, and associations, largely dependent on the teacher involved, and the politics of the day. What is "traditional" is a subject of much debate even within each school.

Three figures have come to be known as the fathers of the modern martial arts: Gichin Funakoshi (*karate-do*), Jigoro Kano (*judo*), and Morihei Ueshiba (*aikido*). Their influence has been considerable, and remarkable in the extent to which so many of the current disparate schools find their way back somehow to one of these individuals. Nevertheless, it would be an injustice to many great teachers neglected by the need to simplify the histories, to see them as the only masters of martial arts as we know them today. While many true masters were content to teach in their homes or on the village square, and in fact found it necessary to stay small in scope to prevent dilution or distortion of their teachings, others labored long and hard to spread the knowledge of martial arts to other lands and cultures.

The modern Korean and Japanese lines of martial arts were introduced to North and South America, and by extension Europe, primarily as a result of the Second World War and the Korean War. Although there were small numbers of practitioners outside of Asia before this time, the arts of the various schools went unrecognized to a great degree until their teachers fled conflict or its aftermath in their homelands. Leaving behind family and homes in countries where the study of martial arts was strictly banned, many came to America and began to teach returning servicemen. Some of the practices which we think of today as traditional, such as militaristic commands and minimal use of words, only reflected the situation, language limitations, and cultural differences of these early teachers. These newcomers faced difficult challenges in trying to teach complex techniques and sophisticated and subtle philosophical ideas to a society unaware of them. Their students who learned in this manner have passed it on in a similar way.

Eventually, many martial artists organized demonstrations and tournaments that included board and brick breaking and other crowd pleasing tricks, in an effort to encourage an enthusiasm for martial arts among the general public. Although successful in attracting attention, these demonstrations may have done more harm than good by distorting both the purposes and the methods of the training.

It can be presumed that many of these teachers suffered from racism in their new homes because of their backgrounds, particularly those from countries with which the West had been in conflict so recently. Although clearly impressed with the skills and stamina demonstrated, the reaction in America to something so completely foreign, and the associations with recent militarism and atrocities of war, certainly delayed the popular reception of the martial arts from Asia. At the same time it was natural for Chinese, Japanese, and Korean communities to practice some protective cultural isolation in their new countries, and the martial arts were thought by some to be too valuable to be shared. Ethnocentrism as well has inhibited the transmission of knowledge in both directions.

Modern media, especially film and television, have not been kind in the portrayal of the true nature of martial arts. Prejudice and misunderstanding have played their roles here as well, and martial artists have either been presented as superhuman or played as clowns. Interest in *ninjutsu, wing chun kung fu* and the *jeet kune do* of Bruce Lee have been spurred by movies and popular culture and are often trivialized because of this, although their roots are as sound and traditional as other more respected forms. Unfortunately, these attacks on truth have not come only from the outside. The quality and predictability of martial arts movies produced by the community itself, has played into the hands of those prepared to profit from this circus of illusion.

In the late sixties and early seventies, martial arts experienced a huge surge in popularity. Magazines, television, movies, tournaments and demonstrations spread the message worldwide. Schools of *karate-do* and *kung fu* opened everywhere and cult followings gathered in awe of such action heroes as Billy Jack, Kato, and Kwai Chang Caine. Bruce Lee first came to notice as a basically silent but mobile chauffeur, bodyguard, and sidekick in the TV series *Green Hornet*. He then went on to international stardom in movies, culminating in the box office hit *Enter the Dragon*, released shortly after his death in 1973. *James Bond*, *Batman*, and the *Man From U.N.C.L.E.*, were also incorporating the karate chop in defense against world-threatening evil. The *Kung Fu* TV series was number one on the networks, and managed to bring the non-violent meditative philosophy of the martial arts to the awareness of the general public. As *kung fu* infiltrated the pop culture of the day it was also the subject of ridicule, sometimes with racist undertones. Nevertheless, numerous Hollywood celebrities were quietly drawn to the study of martial arts for fitness, self-defense, and mental serenity. Interviews at the time with these individuals, many of whom were serious students, always stressed the healthful benefits that they experienced.

At the same time that interest in Zen, yoga, meditation, and Eastern philosophy was becoming widespread, the peace movement and a reaction to anything seeming to be violent

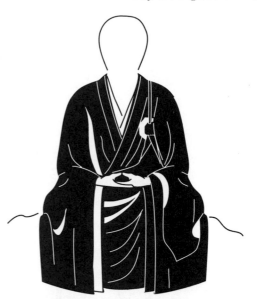

Spiritualism and philosophy permeate the martial arts.

created some sharp contradictions for those teaching martial arts and those who had been or would have been interested in them. Seemingly militaristic practices did not appeal to pacifists and Asian teachers were often scorned and made the butt of racial jokes.

In an attempt to steer the reputation of the martial arts back into the arena of respect, most teachers concentrated on the athletic influences of their arts and fostered their development as sports. Modern American *karate* and full-contact styles have embraced competitive elements, influenced by professional boxing and wrestling in their staging of events and the tournament emphasis on winning. While this has encouraged the spread of schools, and resulted in recognition by sport associations and business interests all the way up to the Olympics, much of the original spirit and philosophical foundations of martial arts have been abandoned by the wayside.

The martial arts have continued to thrive in the eighties and nineties but primarily as sports. Martial arts movies contain much action but little philosophy, and not much information about how the training works to produce results. Even the popular *Karate Kid* movies of the eighties, which spoke directly of the *do* nature of the arts, and the relationship of *sensei* to student, failed to be realistic by turning the scrawny teenager into a tournament-winning fighting hero in six weeks. Since that time, popular movies containing martial arts have tended toward stories of underground tournaments, revenge, or vigilante action. In commercial action movies the violence and special effects have to look very real, and little attention is paid to how the heroes or antagonists acquire their skills, or how their ability manifests itself in other

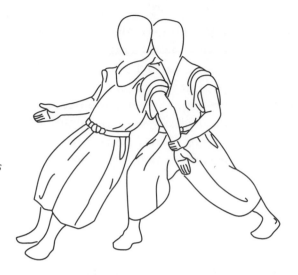

Early practitioners of weaponless techniques trained both for self-defense and exercise.

aspects of their lives. Training and technique tends to be over-exaggerated and sensationalist; where one punch would serve, a jumping spinning kick, landing in the splits, will do much better. But movies are movies, and although fans of most other genres are able to distinguish between entertainment and reality, martial artists are somehow called to answer for these cinematic feats. Unfortunately, few films exist, such as *Iron and Silk*, which eloquently explore the perseverance, sense of learning, and joy of mastery that are embodied in the correct study of martial arts.

The slap-stick humor of martial arts is still reflected in the popular movies of Jackie Chan and the intense interest of young people in the feats of the *Teenage Mutant Ninja Turtles*. The *Power Rangers* and *Mortal Combat* merged the media worlds of TV, movies, and video and arcade computer games and managed to annoy parents, generate millions for their producers, and undermine the hard work of peaceful dedicated martial arts teachers everywhere.

Those who are trying to make a living in the martial arts are faced with unfortunate compromises in remaining true to their profession and traditions rather than giving in to the demands of business promotion and marketing. Participation in the martial arts has risen and fallen in waves throughout their modern history, and the craze of the moment has shifted among different styles. Little emphasis has been paid by the buying public to quality of instruction or the true nature of the training.

The modern craze for *jujutsu* and grappling techniques has similarly sprung from the commercialization of a respected school. The most recent and damaging influence on the public perception of the martial arts is the "no holds barred" tournament, typified by the Ultimate Fighting Challenge. Created as a pay-per-view spectacle that supposedly pits "martial artists" of various styles in fights to unconsciousness or submission, the UFC has developed into a controversial gladiator bloodsport that has been banned in many places. It has been denounced by martial artists and others disgusted by the promotion of violence, aggression, and stupidity.

Clearly, the martial arts have dug themselves a bit of a rut in the popular media, and it is no wonder that the average person is still confused about the reality of those who train, and the myths of those who make money from cheapening of martial arts traditions. The un-initiated do not know where to go for good information. Unfortunately, even today, some of the most reputable martial arts magazines still find themselves carrying ads for "seven-day black belts by mail" and "secret death punches" as well as machines for forcing the legs into the splits.

Things are changing though. Just as there have always been teachers and students of integrity quietly pursuing life-long paths in the martial arts, more recognition is being given to Eastern philosophy and health practices. Professional athletes and coaches have turned to the martial arts for guidance and inspiration to improve their training programs.

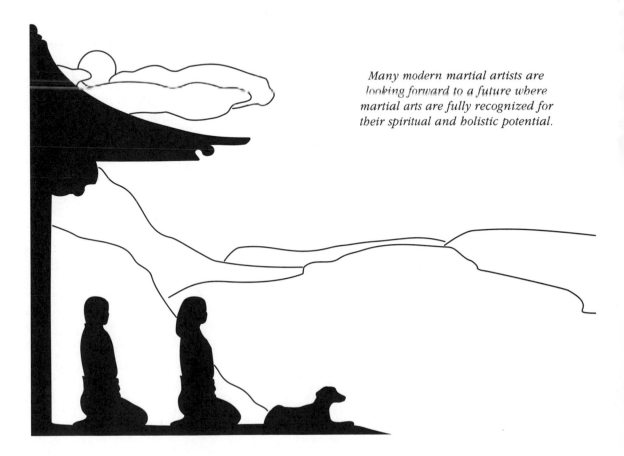

Many modern martial artists are looking forward to a future where martial arts are fully recognized for their spiritual and holistic potential.

They are drawing on the physical, mental, and spiritual aspects of these arts. They are especially interested in how these three are integrated to produce excellence in performance, and how they form a holistic approach to health and fitness, one which can be maintained throughout the life of an athlete. Business seminars and self-help books are based on the strategies and philosophies of both the ancient and modern masters of martial arts. Western medical professionals have begun to open their eyes to a vast corpus of knowledge hidden in those traditions and cultures that have developed separately from those of North America and Europe.

There are many people interested in the martial arts today. Some are admittedly interested primarily in the fighting techniques and the spectator sport aspects, but even they want to know about the physical training. Others are intrigued by the warrior traditions and ethics, the strategies and philosophies. Many are fortunate enough to have discovered for themselves the learning and life-style discipline that good martial arts training has to offer. There are many more who would like to access martial arts knowledge without embracing the whole program, or who need to know more about the health and fitness "secrets" before opening the door to the martial art studio or *dojo*.

It would be incorrect to infer from this brief history of the development of martial arts as we know them today, that the negative aspects are predominant or have occurred only recently. Millions of people worldwide participate in martial arts and most of them practice well, have good teachers, and personally respect the traditions of those who have gone before. Like other disciplines, arts, and professions, there

Martial artists, who take their lessons from nature (and in the case of the authors their canine companions "Sensei" and "Sempai"), do not subscribe to the point of view that humans are highest on the evolutionary scale.

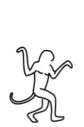 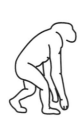 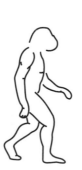 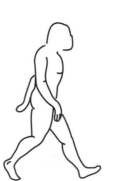 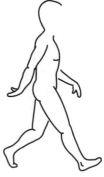

are good and bad examples within the ranks. There have always been changes in emphasis and philosophical debates about the directions to be taken along the path. Historically, the politics of association and business in the martial arts has developed like most group human endeavors, with both strong and weak leadership, and waves of progress and stagnation. Nonetheless, because of the traditions, integrity of instruction, and the profoundly beneficial content of the teachings, martial arts continue to grow in popularity and understanding.

In society at large we have recently seen a growth of interest in things spiritual, and more people taking control of their own health. Holistic treatments, alternative healing practices, and the influences of "new age" beliefs are changing popular culture and consumer buying patterns. It may well be that modern society has come to need what martial arts have to offer to individuals, and by extension, their communities.

The history of martial arts is one of cross-pollination, changing allegiances, interrupted lines, and divergent points of view. However, many fine traditions embodying excellence, respect, and integrity have survived and blossomed in modern times. Some schools have maintained or attempted to return in new ways to traditional roots. Their goal is to obtain the benefits to health, spirit, and character that the martial arts have to offer, to those prepared for a deep study of "the Way." We may need to draw on these sources of ancient knowledge to overcome current trends toward stress, conflict, and illness, and turn them toward peace and health in the future. The long journey that is the path of human progress has always been one of measured, incremental steps.

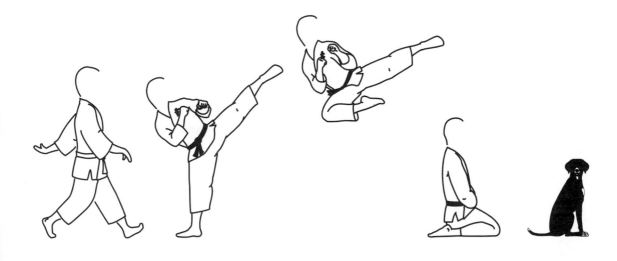

Secrets of the Martial Arts

- What sets the martial arts apart from most exercise systems is their stress on the integration of the mind with the body.

- It is said that Bodhidharma visited the Shaolin temple and taught the monks techniques for breathing and meditation, along with exercises for health and self-defense.

- Respect for elders and the relationship of a student to a *sensei* (literally, "one who has gone before") is an important concept that has influenced the transmission of martial arts knowledge. Another fundamental concept is that of the *tao* (in Chinese; *do* in Japanese), loosely defined as the Way, a philosophical approach that emphasizes self-improvement.

- In trying to understand the influence of martial history on modern schools, one must distinguish between the training and accomplishments of armies for organized warfare, and the individual preparations, attitudes, and achievements of the classical warrior.

- Most of the popularly recognized forms of martial art such as *karate-do*, *judo*, *aikido*, *taekwondo*, etc., have been created in the last hundred years.

- Modern media, especially film and television, have not been kind in the portrayal of the true nature of martial arts. Prejudice and misunderstanding have played their roles here as well, and martial artists have either been presented as superhuman or played as clowns.

- Professional athletes and coaches have turned to the martial arts for guidance and inspiration to improve their training programs. They draw on the physical, mental, and spiritual aspects of these arts.

- Because of the traditions, integrity of instruction, and the profoundly beneficial content of the teachings, martial arts continue to grow in popularity and understanding.

- The history of martial arts is one of cross-pollination, changing allegiances, interrupted lines, and divergent points of view.

Chapter 2

The Simple Act of Breathing

EACH breath we take, from the first to the last, is the very measure of our days.

Continuously, we engage in an exchange with the air around us. Our organism replenishes its supply of oxygen and rids itself of carbon dioxide through the process of respiration.

Breathing is unusual as a bodily function. Unlike most other vital processes (the pumping of the heart, the filtering of the kidneys, for example, where the body continues performing the process unconsciously), we also have a voluntary control over breathing rhythms and volumes. We can hold our breath to go underwater, exhale to sing a long sustained tone, or inhale a deep lungful of scented air in a pine forest. This is an important area in the distribution of power between the body and the mind; neither is in complete control and the balance is always subject to negotiation.

Why then, do we tend to completely ignore our breathing? Unless congested with flu or out of breath after climbing a long flight of stairs, we hardly take notice of our most vital activity.

The martial artist, however, studies this delicate relationship as a fundamental of training. He practices with careful attention to breathing in order to energize and efficiently utilize the body's power. By consciously controlling his exhalations, he can calm the mind and relax emotional responses.

Although we all breathe, we don't all breathe very well. For many, the modern sedentary lifestyle rarely compels us to breathe deeply or rapidly unless we are stressed or angry. Running to the bus stop can put some people out of breath and it is often at these times that one thinks: "Oh, I've got to get in shape!" Even for those already committed to a fitness lifestyle, going for a walk or run along streets congested by the internal combustion engine and construction dust can do more damage than good to the lungs and immune systems.

There are several important considerations regarding improving one's breathing. One is capacity, the actual volume of air that can enter and leave the lungs. Another is the aerobic ability of the system. What is most important about both of these is the actual efficiency of the gaseous exchange going on in the alveoli, the thin vessels deep in the lungs across whose membranes the molecules of oxygen and carbon dioxide enter and leave the bloodstream. This movement and circulation represent the real capacity of breathing to energize, replenish, and refresh the body as a whole.

In practicing both Zen and the martial arts, it is essential to concentrate on breathing out.

•

Taisen Deshimaru
1914–82

Early in their training martial artists will learn to inhale and exhale in such a way that maximum gas exchange can take place at the cellular level. Greater control over the mechanism of breathing can benefit technique, timing, and the overall health and strength of the body. Through abdominal breathing, muscles can be alternately contracted and relaxed to maximize breathing potential and provide anatomical support to the body. Expanding the mind's ability to focus and empty in the same way, is an additional benefit of the exercise of breathing.

Emphasis is placed on the slow exhalation phase of the breathing. This promotes the full emptying of the lungs of waste by-products but also prolongs the time that the body is in the exhalation mode. Studies and practice have shown that one is stronger for pushing, pulling, striking, jumping, etc., when breathing out, especially if the breath can be controlled to assist in the timing of an event. Absorbing a blow or maintaining balance is aided by breath control, and an audible shout or *kiai* is often utilized at the moment of maximum strength or impact.

When frightened or anxious we tend to inhale more rapidly, and holding the breath when startled is common. However, the body's muscle strength drops rapidly when a breath is held, and the consequent buildup of carbon dioxide in the blood and brain triggers more anxiety and fatigue. Hyperventilation or uncontrolled shallow gasping for breath can completely short circuit the timing of the breathing mechanism, and bring about a response close to panic.

The martial artist learns to breathe from the abdomen in a manner similar to yoga practitioners, singers, actors, and wind instrument players. This is also referred to as breathing from the diaphragm. Both these descriptions are misleading because, of course, all breathing is done with the lungs, but as a mental image, the idea of centering the breath low in the body is helpful in retraining the breathing response.

Children and animals at rest naturally breathe with visible movement of their abdomens, rather than their chests. Adult humans seem to have lost this natural ability, and we can only speculate on the cause. The ideal body image in the West demands a flat abdomen and well-developed upper body, and fashions which are worn tightly about the waist and hips only help to constrict the breathing. Too much sitting in desk chairs, television couches, and automobiles has certainly debilitated our posture; combined with very little cardiovascular demand for oxygen in these positions, this has likely contributed to shallowness of breathing (and thinking too, one might argue).

It is believed that to strenghten the spirit, it is essential to strengthen the abdomen.

•

Masutatsu Oyama

1923–94

Although a large volume of air will enter the nose and mouth when we take a big breath, only a small portion of this air will travel as far as the alveoli. This is particularly true if the breath we take is shallow and the lungs are not fully inflated. Many people breathe only with the upper portion of their lungs even when engaged in an activity that demands a good oxygen supply. A visible indicator is the extent that the shoulders rise and fall while breathing. The chest cavity is looking for room to expand and shoulder movement will result. This is not, however, the best way to improve capacity, as it still confines the air exchange to a small portion of the upper lungs. In order to answer the oxygen demands of the body, the rate of respiration (number of breaths per minute) will increase. Normally, this compensation does not nearly fulfill the potential available.

Martial artistis, on the other hand, work to control their breathing and expand the capacity of the lungs by strengthening and localizing the response of the diaphragm muscle, in order to allow expansion of the lung tissue down into the abdominal cavity.

The diaphragm is a smooth, thin sheet of muscular tissue that stretches in a double dome shape from back to front across the body, completely separating the thoracic cavity (which holds the heart and lungs) from the abdomen (intestines, stomach, liver, etc.). When we inhale deeply, the diaphragm works to push gently against the abdominal organs, pulling down the pleural cavity around the lungs. The lower ribs swing outward and upward to allow the lung tissue to expand downward into the space created. Most texts on physiology look upon the act of inhalation as the part of ventilation that requires muscular effort and

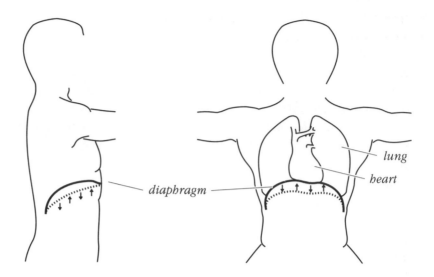

diaphragm

lung

heart

the expenditure of energy. From their point of view, it is exhalation that is the automatic and relaxation phase of the muscles involved. Martial artists and others interested in working with the body's breathing mechanism as a tool, train their "instrument" to be used in just the opposite manner. They consider exhalation the working or power phase, with inhalation occuring to restore the relative atmospheric pressure.

Taisen Deshimaru, a prominent Zen master, emphasizes in *The Zen Way to the Martial Arts* the importance of breathing out slowly, with control and always from the abdomen. He maintains that it is vital to good health to train using *zazen* (seated meditation) to make this response unconscious, so that it can be performed when sleeping as well as when physically active. In addition to the calming effect on the mind and the release of tension in the upper body, it is important for the martial artist to realize that he should strike only when breathing out, and guard against the vulnerability of the moment of inhalation, a weak point in any defense.

This inhalation can be especially dangerous for the martial artist who is not breathing from the abdomen, or *hara*. An intake of breath that is too "upward" in the body redirects the attention away from a low, stable center of gravity, and can be all an opponent needs to knock you off balance. Receiving a blow to the chest or abdomen when inhaling can have the disastrous effect of disabling the breathing signal mechanisms, familiarly known as "having the wind knocked out of you." Exhalation during a blow and the accompanying tensing of abdominal muscles reduces this effect and protects vital organs.

Striking as an opponent inhales is a simple counterattack skill. Learning to read this intention in others is facilitated by observing one's own breathing, balance, and body language. Even a simple signal such as the flaring of nostrils before an attack gives away the breathing rhythm of the opponent, and watching carefully can reveal a need for oxygen. Movement of the shoulders or chest can telegraph the intention to strike and can be used to fake the start of a technique. As part of the study of tactics, a student of *ninjutsu*, popularly known as a *ninja*, learns to breath silently and without motion of the body for stealth and "invisibility." The warrior, combatant, or competitor learns to syncopate the breathing rhythm to confuse opponents, preventing them from taking advantage of vulnerabilities.

Other metabolic systems of the body are influenced by respiration even if they are not directly controlled by ventilation. The lymphatic immune system operates in the body fighting invading diseases, and although not yet completely understood, its circulation has been shown to be strongly affected by breathing processes. It is postulated that contraction of abdominal muscles suppresses the sympathetic nervous system, having the result of reducing common reactions to stress and fear (increased heart rate and blood pressure), allowing some measure of control over emotional reactions. The autonomic nerve center of the solar plexus is also affected by abdominal breathing. This network controls the digestive processes and waste removal mechanisms of the liver and kidneys by controlling the circulatory ability of small blood vessels and capillaries.

Yoga has a long legacy of belief in and practice of the detoxification and purification of body, mind, and spirit by breathing technique. *Chi kung, tai chi chuan,* and *shiatsu* are Asian healing practices that teach breathing as a fundamental basis for self-healing or the treatment of others. Modern movement therapies such as Feldenkrais, Alexander, Trager Mentastics, and Rolfing all have accessed this ancient knowledge for their exercises that coordinate breathing and physical action to improve health.

What then is this abdominal or diaphragmatic breathing? What does it feel like and how is it obtained? Many teachers describe the physical process of letting your abdomen rise (when you are in a horizontal position) or extend, keeping the chest still. Many beginners find this difficult to achieve as they fill their upper lungs first, and then try to "stick their stomach out." Learning to engage the diaphragm consciously is the key to this type of breathing.

If we imagine the body cavity as a vessel to be filled with air rather than water, we can visualize pouring the air right to the bottom and the level rising as it fills. Even more helpful, (and anatomically correct), is a mental image of a balloon with a bulgy bottom that inflates at the base and expands spherically outward in all directions. This expansion is lightly controlled by tension in the abdomen and by

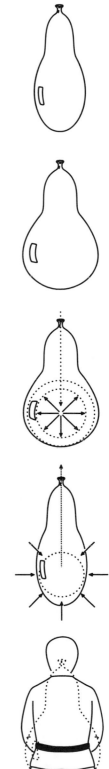

maintaining proper alignment of the pelvis, spine, and head. Feeling that the expansion is occurring across the lower back helps properly position the abdominal cavity, and is part of the therapeutic value of utilizing breathing exercises to those working with body mechanics.

Another factor in how the "balloon" is filled, is the shaping of the oral and nasal cavities. The opening and closing of the mouth, holding the teeth clenched, or engaging the soft palate will affect the pressure of the air and the nature of its passage both in and out of the lungs.

Breathing passively and quietly through the nose will usually engage only the upper area of the lung, indicated by chest rising and often the shoulders lifting as well. In exhalation, by closing slightly the soft palate at the back of the nose and throat, a gentle resistance pressure is created at the exit, which both strengthens the diaphragm muscle and allows for control over the movement of air through the passages. If you think of swallowing or closing the back of the nose when underwater you can close the soft palate. Relaxing the abdominal contraction and then inhaling with open and relaxed throat, will allow the lungs to expand downward, the abdomen expand outwards, and at most we should see the lower floating ribs move with the inhalation and exhalation.

In *zazen* meditation, the martial artist will concentrate on breathing with a slow measured exhalation. By sitting in *seiza* (a kneeling

Zen Testing

EXPERIMENTS on Zen monks have documented the physiological effects of *zazen* breathing on circulation, ventilation, metabolism, and brain wave patterns. Tests were done using a respiratory pneumograph for a comparison of thoracic versus abdominal breathing, a Douglas bag to analyse gas exchange, and electroencephalographs to monitor brain activity.

It was clear in most studies that participants who had more experience, many years of training in abdominal breathing and meditation, displayed consistent results and more control over the body's processes even when subject to testing distractions and interruptions. In general, the tests have shown that once *zazen* breathing has been established, the number of breaths per minute drops dramatically, along with oxygen consumption, to well below normal levels. At the same time, contrary to what was predicted, there was no change in the blood oxygen concentration, thereby indicat-

ing that the oxygen and carbon dioxide exchange became more efficient due to increased tidal volume and metabolic changes.

The reports also remarked on the apparent ability of breath regulation to impart a physiological and psychological control over emotional responses due to the relationship of the autonomous nervous system and the control center of mental processes.

Other studies have shown the positive results of utilizing the *zazen* exercises as therapeutic techniques in the treatment of a variety of physical and psychological disorders.

Sources:
- *Oriental Breathing Therapy*
  by Takashi Nakamura
- *Psychological Studies on Zen*
  by Yoshiharu Akishige
- *Zen Training, Methods and Philosophy*
  by Katsuki Sekida
- *Zen Meditation and Psychotherapy*
  by Tomio Hirai, M.D.

position with the spine straight, shoulders and head relaxed, and arms resting comfortably), the student can become more mentally aware of the rhythms of breathing, and the expansion and contraction of the upper body to accommodate the ventilation process.

This exercise is often practised at the beginning and end of martial art classes as a quiet moment to compose oneself and prepare mentally for the training. The breathing exercise aids in this calming effect. But the principle reason for *zazen*, especially for beginning martial artists, is to train the breathing mechanism, first consciously and then unconsciously, so that during the more energetic phases of the training, they will still be breathing smoothly and efficiently without having to devote much attention to the process. At more advanced levels of training, *zazen* meditation provides other benefits, which will be discussed in later chapters.

There are many different ways of breathing, depending on the position and activity of the body. In martial arts, as in *zazen* breathing, the emphasis is on the abdominal exhalation, yet the pattern of breaths will vary. Particularly in the more vigorous phases of training the intake and expiration of air can be fast or slow, silent or noisy, with tension or relaxation, depending on the requirement of the technique and the task at hand. What is important is the voluntary control of the breathing at the center of the movement, rather than the breathing response limiting what the body and the mind want to do. This is not to say that technique should not flow from the breathing, as this is a fundamental of graceful, strong movement in any activity. But the martial artist trains to strike a balance between the physiological demands of the organism and the intention of the spirit and mind, to best utilize the body's energy and dynamic resources to achieve its goal.

As we naturally emit a grunt or groan when lifting a heavy object, in the same way a martial artist will focus the exhalation of air with a vocal sound into a *kiai*. The word itself means union of spirit energy, from the Japanese for *ki* (energy) and *ai* (union), and therefore represents more than the mere physical manifestation of a shout. For the martial artist in action the term "spirit yell" best describes the source and meaning of the *kiai*. It is the outward expression and extension of one's internal energy in union with the body and its external surroundings. The breath is believed to be at the center of this energy, which is both spiritual and physical.

In Eastern philosophy, the intrinsic energy of the body is considered to be centered in the hara or *tanden* (an area just below and behind the navel). It is essential that the *kiai* be formed from air expelled from the deepest area of the lungs and controlled by the abdominal muscles. The *kiai* will take on many forms, as will be discussed later, depending on the task or flow of the moment, such as pulling, pushing, entering, and turning. A sharp exhalation *kiai* is used by martial artists to accompany short percussive strikes, blows, or blocks.

Sanchin breathing practice, most often associated with the *goju-ryu* and *uechi-ryu* styles of Okinawan *karate-do* (originally from the *pangai-noon* style of Chinese *kempo* and thought by some to be the original lessons given by Bodhidharma to the Shaolin monks) is used for developing pushing and pulling technique. The air and energy is mustered up in the *hara* and then expelled slowly and gutturally with a slight closure of the soft palate at the back of the throat to control the flow of air. It develops great power and emphasizes rootedness and sturdiness, with energy flowing upward from the ground like a tree standing in a storm. The moving tension of the arms and legs forms an isometric pressure zone around the abdominal cavity, allowing the strengthening of the entire body, and developing the use of this strength in a very controlled manner.

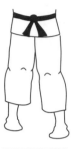

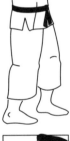

Foot placement for the sanchin-dachi *(three-point stance) for breathing practice, shown in front and side view.*

In striking and grappling techniques, students are often taught to visualize energy "flowing like water through a hose" in conjunction with their exhalation of air, or to "breathe through their hands." Breathing exercises, focus on abdominal contraction and the controlled exhalation of the breath during the performance of techniques is central to the daily training in the martial arts.

After the period of *seiza* at the beginning of a typical class or individual workout, the martial artist will do a series of exercises as a warm-up. The purpose of this is to raise the body temperature so that muscle and connective tissue will stretch and contract without damage. Breathing deeply can boost metabolism and activate energy stored in the chemical systems in the body. It is also important that the mental attitude and breathing rhythm from the *zazen* meditation be carried over into the warm-up, as it is here that the coordination of breathing and physical movement will be established and synchronized. The gentle stretches and rotations done to limber and loosen the joints and spine will be performed with slow exhalation, taking care to not hold the breath. If done correctly and with attention to the pattern and depth of breathing, a nice flowing movement of the body will result, and provide a good transition to the vigorous and demanding exercises to follow.

Basic exercises, or *kihon*, can encompass a wide range of techniques practised in combination. These exercises are repeated rhythmically as learning drills for accuracy, strength, stamina and endurance. In *gorin-do*, *karate-do*, *taekwondo*, and others, they can be performed either standing or moving back and forth across the floor or ground. In the throwing and grappling arts of *aikido* or *judo* the pattern of practice with partners may appear to be somewhat different, but the purpose of *kihon* to break down technique into component parts and then rebuild repetitively is the same.

Kihon is excellent training for the improvement of vital capacity, cardiovascular efficiency, and overall fitness and coordination. The closest parallel in conventional physical education is the aerobics exercise class of modern fitness clubs. In fact, the most recent trend in physical fitness training is the incorporation of martial arts and boxing techniques in these classes. Although martial art professionals are happy to see some recognition of the systems that they have been training in for decades, there is concern that there may be insufficient attention being paid to proper preparation and precise technique in order to avoid injury. While they do popularize the whole-body benefits that martial arts training can offer, without the mental and spiritual influence and the grounding in the breathing practices, these exercises provide to participants only a small part of the total "package."

Kihon provides a good aerobic workout in which the mind is always engaged, focusing on accurate technique, breaking it down into parts, recombining, making movements flow with the breath. In more advanced martial arts training, intensive and long training sessions are designed for improving endurance, concentration, and reliance on correct technique to conserve energy. Here the body will pass from aerobic respiration (where oxygen is used directly) to anaerobic respiration, where lactic acid is formed in the muscle tissue and extended feelings of fatigue, both physical and mental, set in. All forms of long distance or endurance exercise will engage the aerobic/anaerobic crossover effect. Good instruction and training can increase the time spent operating aerobically and considerably reduce the discomfort of the anaerobic metabolism. Although the physical effects of the body's "changing of gears" are very real, the reaction to them and their influence on enjoyment and the desire to continue training, or

Now and again, it is necessary to seclude yourself among deep mountains and hidden valleys to restore your link to the source of life. Breathe in and let yourself soar to the ends of the Universe; breathe out and bring the cosmos back inside. Next, breathe up all the fecundity and vibrancy of the earth. Finally, blend the breath of heaven and the breath of earth with that of your own, becoming the Breath of Life itself.

•

Morihei Ueshiba
1883–1969

more to the point, the *perception* of the ability of the body to continue, is largely mental.

The martial artist is working to recognize and control this mind-body effect and use it to his advantage. Understanding and control of breathing is critical in being able to increase the limits of his physical endurance, and eliminate the anxiety induced when "waiting for that second wind," by making that wind come to him. Breathing fuels the metabolic furnace of the body and affects the production of adrenaline and endorphins. These chemical and hormonal influences produce feelings of well-being, pain relief, and surges of energy and power. A martial artist seeks to access the virtually unlimited potential of the human body and spirit that we see demonstrated in situations in which, for example, a mother has to lift a tree branch off her injured child, or the survivor of a plane crash crosses hundreds of miles of bush to seek rescue. Although the physical limits of most humans appears to be finite, it is often the will to survive and the ability to concentrate one's energies on a single task that sets us apart.

Learning to access and harness the body's intrinsic physical resources, uniting the intellect, will, and passion, is the training goal of the martial artist. By recognizing the equilibrium required, and by studying the ebb and flow of these energies, the student or practitioner can work to direct these skills. At the same time, a martial artist is learning to let go, go with the flow, and allow energy to come to him. This *yin-yang* balance between control and chaos is part of what makes the martial arts so challenging and interesting, both as an activity and a way of life.

Yin and Yang

THIS well-known graphic represents a balanced interplay of pairs of essential but opposing forces, each containing some component of its opposite, thus generating a cyclical, eternal ebb and flow of the activities and qualities of each member of the pair.

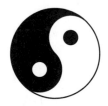

Pairings descriptive of yin *and* yang

push / pull	*salty / sweet*
hard / soft	*control / chaos*
light / dark	*loud / quiet*
in / out	*white / black*
up / down	*heavy / light*

Training in *kata* (a formal series of arranged movements), is the next step in the integration of natural flowing movements and breathing. Fast and slow, push and pull, grappling and jumping are all included in these moving meditations. Initially perceived as a teaching exercise, its role expands as the student progresses. *Kata* is considered by some as the highest form of expression in the martial arts and is certainly where mind, body and spirit come together. Endless repetition of *kata*, "polishing the diamond," allows

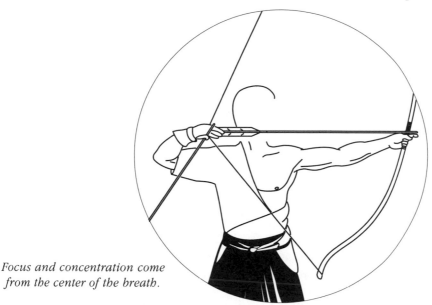

*Focus and concentration come
from the center of the breath.*

students eventually to let go of the mental and physical limitations of the training and breathe with the spirit of the art.

The martial artist is using the breathing process of meditation in extreme moments of excellence or survival. By concentrating on the breathing in various levels of respiration, the brain acquires a focus that can be used to calm the mind or inspire it. Deep breathing can serve to both energize and relax at the same time. Feelings of anxiety that often result from the organism of the body being unsettled or stressed can be quelled, and the effects of adrenaline and other by-products of the body's metabolism can be controlled. As well, emphasizing the benefits of allowing the body to perform in optimum conditions, with a positive attitude, can significantly enhance one's sense of general well-being and happiness. Just learning to relax can release great energy in the body and spirit. The old adage "just take ten deep breaths" to control anger or other emotions comes from this. Through training, the martial artist seeks to become more "present" in every moment. Being aware and engaging fully in the experience at hand is both a philosophical fundamental and a necessity for the martial artist. Communicating and expressing this with the physical senses, always brings us back to how we "breathe in" or absorb our environment, and continuously return energies back to it.

Prana is the Sanskrit word for the energy given off by the movement and flow of living things in our universe, and is often associated with water and earth that is vibrant and alive. Breathing in the spray of waves crashing, waterfalls flowing, and the scent of verdant forests, fields, or jungles, has always brought joy and health to the human spirit. Whether interpreted as complex interactions of molecules of oxygen, hydrogen, nitrogen, and carbon-based life forms, or metaphysically as union with *ki,* this effect is basically what defines our lives as humans. The simple basis of the systems that allow us to exist should humble and amaze us, and the delicacy of the balance required for survival deserves our respect.

Even the trees breathe. It is not just poetic to consider the large remaining jungles and forests as the lungs of our planet. Deforestation caused by humankind is a serious threat to the balance of ecosystems and the quality of the air we breathe. The oxygen supply of this "Spaceship Earth" exists as a very thin skin around a planet of water, rock, and some organic matter. Although we feel the atmosphere is immense around us, even at an altitude of 10,000 feet, the air is appreciably thinner; it becomes difficult to breathe and the adjustment to different concentrations of elements in the air and in the bloodstream can make our organism feel quite unwell.

Breathing problems associated with pollution in urban environments arise not just because particulates in the air are inhaled, but also because of the imbalance of gases and the lack of oxygen-producing plants and trees in these concrete and asphalt environments.

The martial artist not only exercises caution in avoiding polluted air, but constantly seeks out opportunities to fill his lungs and spirit with

Breathing Attitudes

M ARTIAL arts breathing is a singular symbiosis of "laughing" and "coughing." Both mechanisms are employed to clean and activate the whole self, from the inside out.

	LAUGHING	COUGHING
Inhale	*Short*	*Long*
Exhale	*Long*	*Short*
The body	*Limbs externalized (clapping and stamping on the floor)*	*Bend forward and raise the back to contract the abdomen muscles (internalized)*
Benefits	*Activates circulatory system Induces relaxation*	*Cleans respiratory apparatus Promotes contraction*
Attitude	*Open*	*Closed*
Senses	*Open*	*Closed*
Application	*Striking, jumping, spinning*	*Grappling, anchoring, pulling*

clean oxygenated and energized air. It is as vital to the feeding and function of the organism as food and water. Protecting the air supply on both an individual and global level is just basic self-defense.

Many martial arts are practised outdoors in a natural environment. Although it is obvious that "unlimited ceiling" assists the practice of weapons technique such as that of *kyudo, kendo, iaido* as well as the staff and stick work of *karate-do, gorindo, aikido* and *kali*, it is the physiological, psychological, and philosophical effects of breathing deeply the natural air and energy that are being studied and utilized. Extending the reach of one's control by "breathing out" through the hands, and then through the ends of the tools or weapon, is a fundamental of these techniques. Strength, finesse, and flow are acquired through such practice.

Fu: *wind, or breath*

Other Japanese arts that employ smaller implements, such as calligraphy, brush painting, and the tea ceremony, are also taught as extensions of the mind and breath. *Zazen* breathing is used to prepare the mind and reflexes and then every movement in the practice arises and flows from the exhalation of the breath. The stroke of the brush on paper or the whisking of the brush in tea is the same as the slice of the blade of the samurai sword; it is the single breath of the artist.

Knowledge and attitudes about breathing are one of the main areas of divergence between Western and Eastern ways of thinking, both culturally and historically. Western science took a very long time to recognize that germs and poisons could invade the body through inhalation. Interest in the conscious control of breathing mechanisms or its connection to personal health is almost conspicuous by its absence. Medical study of ventilation and respiration appears confined to clinical analysis of the human organism and its diseases. Resuscitation and artificial respiration are means of sustaining life, but little analysis of the importance of maintaining breathing as a useful tool of the body, or as an extension of the human mind and spirit has been done in modern Western culture. Perhaps historically the religious fundament to our social and artistic patterns did not allow for "the holy spirit" to be associated with such mundane and profane human processes as breathing. Even though the "heart" has been allowed to embody emotions and will, we don't often expose its true simple function as an oxygen pump for a metabolic furnace. How our conscious thoughts and unconscious memories inhabit this physical machine is still mostly a mystery to the Western paradigm. The Eastern philosophies, religions, medicines, and educational systems, on the other hand, place breathing as a physical process and life force. It has a place as the fundamental point of departure for study, teaching, expression, and understanding of all important Ways. Having good *hara* is as much as assessment of character and integrity as it is a physical and health statement.

Emotionally, the martial artist observes responses to different circumstances that affect the breathing responses unconsciously. Through *zazen* and martial arts training the student can learn to reverse the roles, making the breathing patterns influence thoughts and create new situations. Adjusting one's attitude can be reduced to exhaling the old completely and welcoming the new.

Life and death is the philosophical paradigm for the influence of the samurai tradition on the martial arts. Each cycle of breathing is a day-night unit in an organism, a *yin-yang* cellular life unit. From a psychological and philosophical point of view, the experience of "living in the moment" can be defined as the duration of a breath, a "mini-life." This influence of Zen upon the character of martial arts and those who study the Way helps the organism and the person obtain full value for life. By enjoying each breath you take, life becomes long, fruitful, and healthy, the ultimate goals of the martial artist.

Putting the Ball on the Shelf
Gorindo Breathing Exercise No. 1

Basic: Begin in a relaxed, standing position, feet shoulder width apart, and knees loose. Step forward with the right foot into a *sanchin-dachi* (three-point stance, see page 22). Feel the heels pointing slightly to the outside, pelvis pulled under and tilting up, knees pushing gently (without discomfort) to the inside, creating three points of a stable triangle.

Inhale while raising the hands in front of the solar plexus, keeping elbows tucked in and ensuring the shoulders are down and relaxed. Pause briefly to balance the relaxation and tension. Begin exhaling with a very slight pressure upon the air in the throat with the soft palate and slowly direct the hands upward and away from the body to the level of the face, *jodan.*

Feel the abdomen contract, the shoulders drop, and the pelvis pull underneath at the end of the exhalation. Pause. Maintain that alignment of the body, and bring hands back again to the solar plexus while inhaling. The next breath is exhaled as you push hands directly forward from and to the solar plexus level, *chudan.* Bring the hands back again with the inhalation and then exhale, pushing downward and away from the body to the level of the *hara* (just below the navel), *gedan.* Retrieve the hands on an inhalation back to the solar plexus and relax, exhaling as the hands drop to the sides.

The second half of the exercise repeats with the other foot forward.

Intermediate: Step forward at the same time as inhaling and raising hands. Step back with exhalation while dropping hands. More pressure can be used against the closing of the palate.

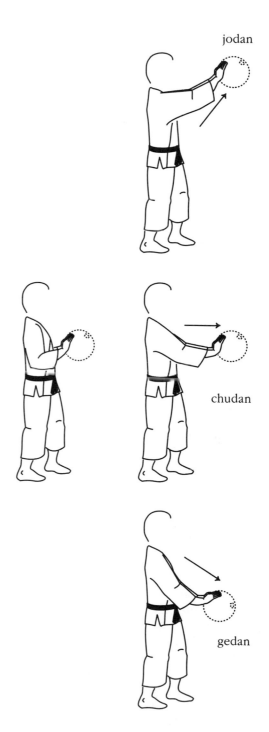

jodan

chudan

gedan

Casting Petals to the Winds
Gorindo Breathing Exercise No. 2

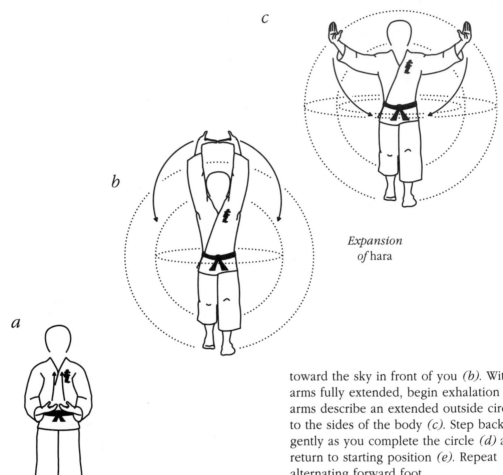

c

b

a

Expansion of hara

Basic: Stand with feet together, hands palm up, fingertips together in front of you, cradling your *hara* or *ki* center just below your navel *(a)*. With a gentle rocking motion, step forward while bringing your hands up the center of your body as you inhale. As your hands pass the level of your face rotate them to a palms up and thumbs up position, then push upward toward the sky in front of you *(b)*. With arms fully extended, begin exhalation as arms describe an extended outside circle to the sides of the body *(c)*. Step backward gently as you complete the circle *(d)* and return to starting position *(e)*. Repeat alternating forward foot.

Intermediate: Push and tense with isometric pressure at the closing of the circle as you return hands to center. Try to feel that you are describing a sphere with your body, breath, and mind. Take care that your eyes look forward and upward on the extension but without your head falling back onto the neck. The rocking motion of the step involves walking heel first and then shifting the weight to the ball of the foot as the heel of the trailing foot lifts off the ground. To return, reverse the process. Proceed with the motions without stopping in between.

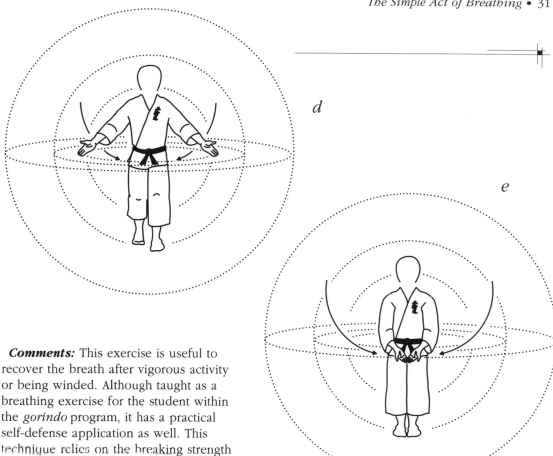

d

e

Comments: This exercise is useful to recover the breath after vigorous activity or being winded. Although taught as a breathing exercise for the student within the *gorindo* program, it has a practical self-defense application as well. This technique relies on the breaking strength achieved from the exhalation of air and can be used to defend from a double wrist grab, or in this case, a front choking grab. The defender steps into the opponent, raises hands in front and above, and exhales as hands move in an outward circle, breaking the hold and, if desired, trapping the opponent's arms under his own as he completes the lower portion of the circular movement.

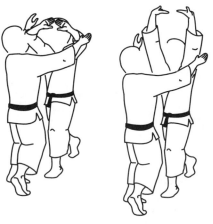

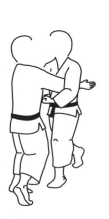

The Archer's Bow (standing or kneeling)
Gorindo Breathing Exercise No. 3

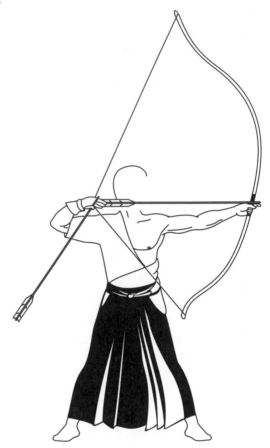

Basic: Begin with hands and shoulders relaxed, palms up. Raise hands slowly in front as you inhale, keeping the shoulders down and letting the abdomen relax and expand. Move the head and arms to the left, describing a circle with the eyes moving with the hands, exhaling slowly and fully contracting your abdomen as you complete the drawing of the bow. At the release of the string, release the tension in the abdomen, relax the throat, and allow the air to refill from the bottom of your lungs as if you are the target attracting the arrow. Follow the air with the sweep of the arms back to center. Begin to exhale again when the hands are together in front of the chest and allow your hands to return slowly to the lap. Breathe normally for a breath or two, then repeat on the other side.

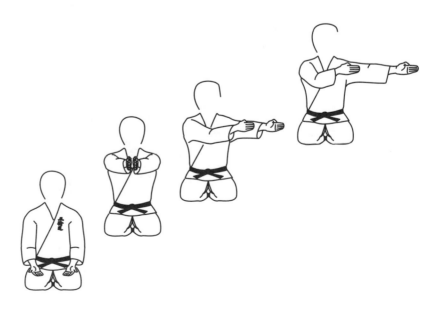

Intermediate: The mechanics of the movement are the same but as a physical and mental exercise, the dynamic of the breathing changes.

Raise hands in front. Continue to inhale as your hands draw to the side. As the near pulling hand begins to cross the expanding (but not rising) chest, a slight pause or retention of the breath occurs without pressure. As the arrow is "released," follow the return of the hands with an exhalation downward into the abdomen. Remember that the visualization of the inhalation and exhalation occurs not just to fill the area of vision in front of you, but describes a semicircle behind you as well. By repeating the movements on the other side of the body, you should create a mental image of concentric circles with yourself as the eye of the target.

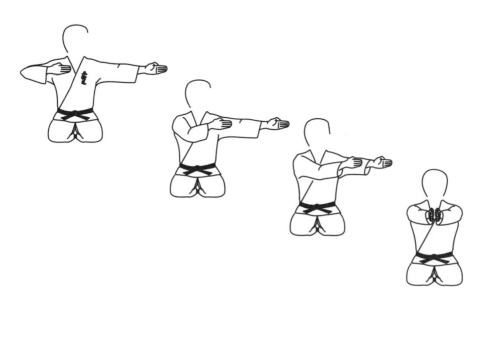

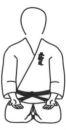

Secrets of the Martial Arts

- Early in their training martial artists learn to inhale and exhale in such a way that maximum gas exchange can take place at the cellular level. Greater control over the mechanism of breathing can benefit technique, timing, and the overall health and strength of the body.

- Emphasis is placed on the exhalation phase of breathing. This promotes the full emptying of the lungs of waste by-products and also prolongs the time that the body is in the exhalation mode.

- Martial artists work to control their breathing and expand the capacity of the lungs by strengthening and localizing the response of the diaphragm muscle.

- It is essential that the *kiai* be formed from air expelled from the deepest area of the lungs and controlled by the abdominal muscles.

- It is important that the mental attitude and breathing rhythm from the *zazen* meditation be carried over into the physical warm-up, as it is here that the coordination of breathing and physical movement will be established and synchronized.

- Although the physical effects of the body's "changing of gears" are very real, the *perception* of the ability of the body to continue is largely mental. Martial artists work to recognize and control this mind-body effect and use it to their advantage.

- Endless repetition of *kata*, "polishing the diamond," allows students eventually to let go of the mental and physical limitations of the training and breathe with the spirit of the art.

- Concentrating on the breathing in various levels of respiration allows the brain to acquire a focus that can be used either to calm or to inspire the mind.

- The martial artist not only exercises caution in avoiding polluted air but seeks out opportunities to constantly fill the lungs and spirit with clean oxygenated and energized air.

- The Eastern philosophies, religions, medicines, and educational systems recognize breathing as a physical process and life force.

Chapter 3

Keeping in Line with Your Spine

THE bony spine, and the musculature that allows it to function as it does, is one of several important components of the human body that we mostly ignore until something goes wrong. Then we hear or say: "My aching back!" or "My stiff neck!" and we pay heed only until the pain goes away. However, it is what we do with the spine all the rest of the time that leads to these conditions.

As soon as someone begins to discuss backs, posture, or breathing, we all tend to sit up straighter, pull our shoulders back, and squirm in our chairs. You may well have done so when you began to read this chapter. Although this a good reaction generally, it does indicates that we probably were not sitting or standing properly in the first place. Inactivity, together with poor body positioning does more damage to backs and necks as we age than any vigorous activity such as heavy lifting, tennis serves, or even minor traffic accidents ever could. Although these latter are responsible for many injuries, it is notable that most of the movements that "put the back out" tend to be simple ones like bending too quickly to pick up a sock, reaching over the bed to tuck in a sheet, or lifting a suitcase out of the trunk of your car. What we often fail to realize at these moments is that the fault lies not in the actions themselves, but the neglect to which we have subjected the spinal system for years, and in some cases, whole lifetimes.

Although there are those who have been born with curvatures or anomalies, and others whose injuries have produced conditions that require special care, most of us have allowed our spines to get out of line gradually. Over time, surrounding tissues and muscles have adapted and compensated. Even when told to sit up straight we may feel in

Regions of the Spine

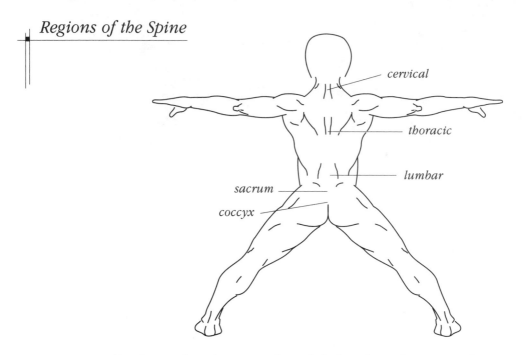

line but in fact there may be subtle bends in the spine. This can cause an unnatural movement of components such as what occurs when your car wheels are out of alignment and the tires wear unevenly. As well, when we age, the spine's natural shock absorbers begin to lose their elasticity, and a severe jolt, especially when vertebrae are twisted out of line, can cause them to fail or break down.

Fortunately, in recent years we have come to recognize, with the help of sports physicians and movement therapists, that these defects can be avoided, and in many cases reversed, by exercise, good posture, and more respect for the framework that supports the body.

The martial artist is already toiling in this field, working away on spinal alignment whether or not he or she has ever experienced back or neck pain before. In much the same way that the students of martial art are trained in the art of breathing, they learn the art of standing and sitting correctly from the very beginning of their practice. In order to move well, the martial artist requires a body that is well tuned and in good running order, one in which reflexes, balance, strength, flexibility, and intrinsic energy are responding in harmony. This is not possible without good alignment of the spine, head, and body.

Since so much martial art training is based on the disciplined and supervised execution of good technique, it offers an excellent opportunity for the development or repair of alignment. Learning the location of your center of gravity and how to lever or rotate the body around it, is practiced from the first day, and continues to a refined subtlety at advanced levels of training. From a health and fitness point of view, elegant technique and feats of balance and agility are all in aid of a relaxed, natural stance.

Developing self-awareness, or a kinesthetic sense of where your various body parts are and how they are moving in the execution of technique, is valuable both in and outside the *dojo*. A martial artist requires the ability to move quickly and change direction, but also to hold his ground in a stable stance when necessary. Although these demands may seem to be contradictory, they are in fact the principles of *yin* and *yang* at work; both are needed for balanced performance.

In the previous chapter about breathing we touched upon the different ideal body images in the East compared with those of the West. The military bearing of the North American phys-ed student calls for broad shoulders, chest thrust out, and gut sucked in. A downward pointed triangle is formed and results in a perceived high center of gravity *(a)*. Gymnastics and ballet also reflect this image of upward mobility. In traditional Eastern movements like the martial arts or dancing, the triangle is reversed, with a wide stable base and lower center of gravity located in the *hara*, in the abdomen *(b)*. To further the analogy, one can see that a pyramid on its point is easily toppled, and while sitting on its base it cannot easily be dragged across the floor. The martial artist learns to stand and move in a way that takes advantage of these principles, building upon the stable foundation or spinning on the tip of the top as needed.

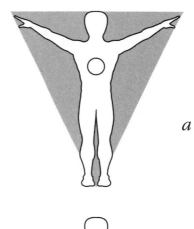

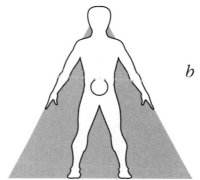

While learning to breathe from the *hara*, the martial art student is also encouraged to "move from the *hara*," feeling the weight low and with the upper body relaxed in motion. Techniques are then taught that allow the upper limbs and upper body to tense and brace upon impact against the rooted foundation *(c)*. Alternatively, being able to spin, turn aside or deflect an attack requires a similar awareness of ground, center of gravity, and rotational axis, but with a relaxed upper body.

The main rotational axis of the body is a line from the center of the head, passing through the body and *hara* and touching the ground at what we could call the center point of the stance. Keeping the

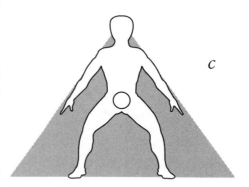

Western (a) and Eastern (b, c) concepts of body image and center of gravity.

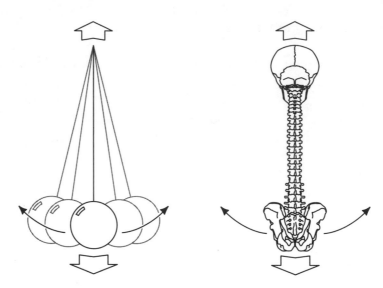

*The pendulum swing of relaxed movement, with the spine
extended in both directions.*

upper body erect and the spine in line permits quick, balanced movement and the application of centrifugal force, using the extended limbs
as striking, blocking, and deflecting weapons. Imagining the cross-sec-
tional plane, the ability to swing like a pendulum in an axis that also
hinges through the *hara*, is valuable for displacement movements and
the utilization of the lower limbs for kicking or sweeping.

The martial artist begins to find his alignment by learning to stand
properly in the "ready" or "natural" position with feet shoulder width
apart, knees unlocked and back pulled up straight as if suspended from
above the head, with the pelvis tucked slightly under. The feet should
feel like they are alive and growing from the ground. Many basic exercises can be performed in this stance so that the student learns the
elements of vertical balance, such as how not to throw weight forward
with a punch that might topple the body.

One of the first things taught to a student entering a Japanese *dojo*
is how to bow from this upright standing position. This is performed
by bringing feet together and bending forward with spine and head in
line dropping to a thirty degree angle (or lower if the respect accorded
by the bow requires it) and returning to the natural stance from this
bow. This is a lesson in *attitude*, both the mental (respect, order, calm-
ness) and the physical (as in the position of an aircraft in relation to a
certain direction or plane).

Next, the student learns how to sit correctly in *seiza* for meditation,
with head and upper body erect, and contemplating his navel or *hara*
(actually a bit below and to the inside of the belly button) as he breathes
from the abdomen.

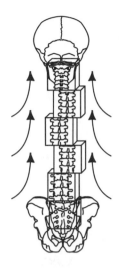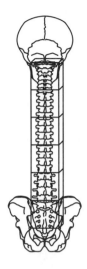

Correct alignment of spinal segments (right) provides structural support and allows smooth movement.

Although the *seiza* position (with head and spine in line) requires some practice and flexibility to achieve, its usefulness in locating the breathing and center of gravity around the *hara* is important. For the beginner, learning to feel the orientation of the body in space, with the eyes closed, is more easily achieved in the *seiza* position than standing, where balance can be compromised.

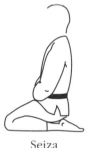

Seiza *position*

Breathing to provide maximum metabolic efficiency also demands a posture that will allow diaphragm movement, and controlled contraction and relaxation of the abdominal muscles. It is interesting to note the relationship of breathing to spinal alignment and how many of the martial arts breathing exercises, when properly performed, actually bring the spine into good alignment as the abdomen expands and reduces the compression of the vertebrae.

In basic *kihon* (fundamental exercise drills), various stances are introduced that move from the natural erect position. Beginning with hands on the hips, the student is able to feel the position of the pelvis and is reminded to keep the weight low for stability. Most martial arts uniforms incorporate a sash, or *obi*, that is worn low on the hips as a further aid to body memory. The traditional Japanese *hakama*, a wide-legged pantaloon, is constructed with a stiff card across the lower back, and is tied in an elaborate fashion across the hips and under the *hara* to provide support for correct posture. As well, the *hakama* reinforces the triangulated stable base image and forces the wearer to move deliberately with the feet and hips.

With well-constructed stances the martial artist will feel himself riding his lower body with an erect, balanced posture. Keeping the head

Major Bones of the Skeleton
(posterior view)

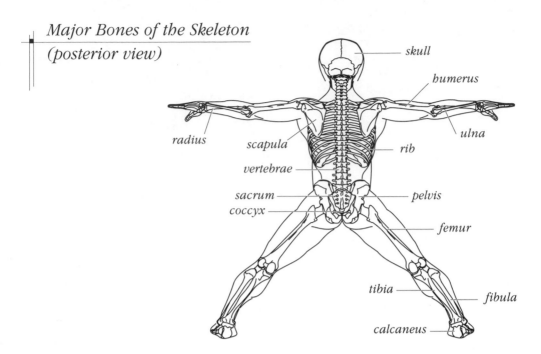

skull

humerus

ulna

radius

scapula

rib

vertebrae

sacrum

pelvis

coccyx

femur

tibia

fibula

calcaneus

poised and in line with the upper spine permits smooth movement when walking or shifting from one stance to the other. Enforcing the discipline of correct posture and technique, "building from the ground up," challenges the patience of the beginning student and teacher alike, but is often what separates the excellent from the merely competent technique as the student progresses. The success of the martial artist in terms of being able to train without injury, and perform increasingly demanding technique, depends on being attentive and dedicated to good form in stances and movement.

The martial artist learns early on that where the head goes, the body will soon follow. The head is a rather heavy ball of brain and bone connected to the body through a narrow channel of muscle, cartilage, and some bony material. If this ball rolls off its pedestal in any direction it tends to pull its base with it. The rest of the spine strains against this unbalancing and creates unnecessary and harmful tension in the body. This can interfere with the technique and impede the body's attempt to properly apply energy.

Relaxed attentiveness is the key to maintaining alignment and proper posture while moving. Learning to sit or stand correctly is a beginning, but of little value if that knowledge cannot be transferred to the body in motion. Progressively introducing new elements of balance such as turning, twisting, standing on one foot, jumping, and so on, allows the martial artist to incorporate the action into a mental awareness of body position. Learning to sense, control, and naturally coordinate the head, neck, hip, and spine requires good instruction and consistent practice.

Most of us (as we engage in the aforementioned squirming in our chair to sit up straight) think that correct posture requires muscular effort and does not feel relaxed. While this may be true for the couch potatoes among us, the martial artist works hard on the conditioning of the body, not just to be able to perform actively, but also for the reward of relaxing without strain, tension, or weakness. In addition, for both the sedentary and the active, consciously sitting, standing, or moving in line will energize the body, awaken the mind, and allow for more focus and endurance when performing tasks. This is of value for those who spend long hours working at a computer, driving, walking a beat, or any routine activity that leads easily to fatigue.

Learning how to strengthen the muscles of the back, abdomen, hips and shoulders to allow for strong movement and correct alignment is a training goal of martial arts. Finding the right balance of relaxation and tension, moving quickly between the two, and localizing those muscles that need to be contracted while others are relaxed, is all part of the repetitive training found in *kihon* practice.

Many modern exercise systems can lead to overdevelopment in one area of the body to the neglect of others, and this can throw our alignment out of true. Bodybuilding, and spot exercises that focus only on attractive muscular appearance, can interfere with flexibility and be a source of repetitive stress injury. Those who have become obsessed with a flat stomach and purchased the latest abdominal exercise contraption can throw their necks or backs out of alignment due to a lack of muscular support, or aggravate problems with discs or vertebrae because of grinding or twisting in bad positions. This is most unfortunate for those who are just beginning an exercise program and have a genuine interest in getting in shape. The tendency to want to make up

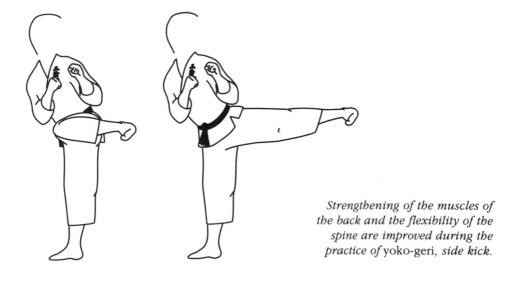

Strengthening of the muscles of the back and the flexibility of the spine are improved during the practice of yoko-geri, *side kick.*

Muscle Groups of the Pelvis
(anterior view)

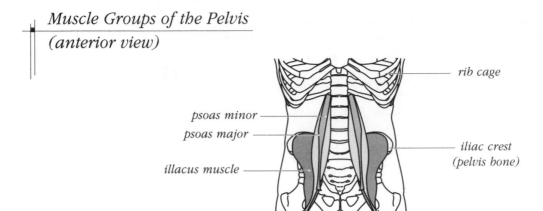

psoas minor

psoas major

illacus muscle

femur

rib cage

iliac crest
(pelvis bone)

quickly for a long period of inactivity contributes to failure. It is important to understand how interconnected the body's muscles, bones, ligaments, and tendons are, and how to train them and correct weaknesses in a gradual way.

Sedentary people have usually let their abdomens sag, and developed lower back pain because the stronger muscles of the back have contracted and tilted the pelvis down and back. Those who are more active, especially runners and cyclists for example, may feel they lack flexibility in their lower back while stretching, when in fact it is the hamstring muscles of the legs that are too tight, inhibiting the ability to bend over to touch the ground. Alignment of the pelvis and hips can often be thrown out of whack by the psoas muscles, which run from the top front of the leg through the hip to the sacrum at the base of the spine. Any of these situations can cause back or neck pain, spinal degeneration, and inhibit mobility, but are technically not conditions of the spine at all. However, long-term imbalance and misalignment can indeed cause serious problems in the spine if not addressed.

Fortunately, there has been a shift away from the traditional medical treatment model of bed rest for back problems. With upwards of eighty percent of Americans suffering lower back pain at some time, supervised exercise has proven to speed dramatically the rate of recovery and prevent the recurrence of acute episodes. These painful seizures can be frightening and are often triggered by simple mistakes. When a nerve has been pinched by a vertebra out of line, or worse, by the pressure of a disc that has bulged or ruptured, the muscles that run the length of the spine will seize and "lock down" to protect the integrity of the spinal column and the essential nerve pathways running inside it. This defense reaction can be much more painful and last longer

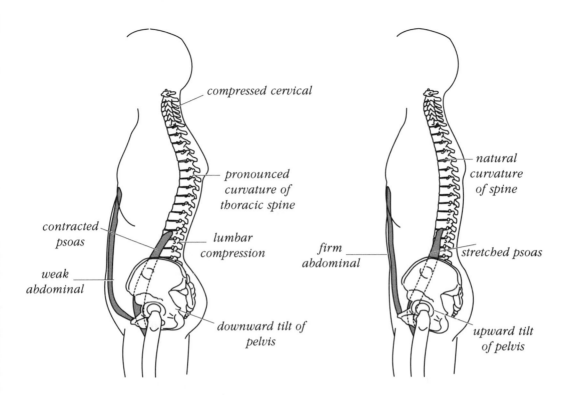

Positions of abdominal and psoas muscles in relation to spine and pelvis.
The left figure illustrates a typically weakened structure contrasted
with correct alignment on the right.

than the injury which caused it. The period of immobilization this causes is often an overreaction on the part of these muscles, but the body takes no chances when it comes to protecting its essential networks.

In the Eastern modality of medicine, most treatment therapies begin with regaining the proper alignment of the spine, and many methods are used to achieve this. *Shiatsu* (digital pressure massage) and *sotai* (gentle manipulation and natural exercise), for example, seek to unlock tension, rebalance the arrangement of muscles and bones, and stimulate vital energy that can aid in healing and supporting the active healthy state. Acupuncture and acupressure also work from the body's natural strengths.

Although martial training is about self-defense and prevention of injury, and does not primarily seek to be a healing art, it can be helpful in the process of recovery from injury after professional diagnosis and treatment. Because martial training incorporates evaluation and self-awareness as well as the feedback of a teacher, it blends particularly well with Eastern health practices. Their emphasis is on the body, mind, and spirit of the whole person as the basis of health, rather than the "treat the illness" point of view often found in Western medicine. Many of the modern alternative movement therapies, such as those of Feldenkrais (himself a *judoka*, the first black belt of Europe), borrow the simple basic exercises found in martial art training and use them, (sometimes slowed or modified for hands-on manipulation), as treatments for illness or injury.

Unless the body is held in accordance with the order of Nature (balanced distribution of the weight without undue muscular strain) compression or suppression is easily brought to bear on its contents, preventing them from conducting their full natural function, thus creating a state of chemical unbalance, the first step towards ill-health.

•

Gunji Koizumi
1885–1965

The field of sports medicine arose to meet the needs of professional athletes and serious recreational enthusiasts. The traditional body of knowledge of the medical establishment had been based on the treatment of sick people, often injured and bed-ridden. Physiotherapy and rehabilitation therapies were seeking to return their patients to normal, but the definitions of the normal condition were based on a statistical average of people who were largely non-athletic. It remains true that to be pronounced "well" or "cured" means simply that a person can go home from the hospital or return to work in a sedentary condition. This is far from satisfactory for the athlete, manual laborer, or in fact any active healthy person such as a martial artist. This is particularly true with regard to neck and back injuries and the range of treatment options available. It is interesting that both chiropractic and osteopathy (the former now more readily accepted by the establishment than the latter), base their training, assessment, and treatment practices on the principle of spinal alignment as the source from which both health and illness can spring.

Martial art training can be recommended as an exercise program because of its supervised, progressive approach, emphasizing good technique and correct body position. Patience, discipline, and an ability to maintain focus in the present moment assist greatly in achieving the benefits of the martial arts exercise regimen. In other sports or activities, participants can become discouraged or forced to quit if the goal orientation or competitive atmosphere does not allow for individual progress within the group. It is important that the teacher be able to assist students in evaluating what is happening with their bodies during the training process.

Some discomfort occurs as a natural process of conditioning the body and adapting it to new movements and capacities. However, pain caused by injury or repetitive stress is an important signal from the body, and should never be ignored. Occasionally, (and particularly true of adult beginners), someone comes to the training with an old injury or condition that has not bothered them when inactive, but rears its ugly head as they begin training. By working in concert with their own health professional, a martial arts student and teacher should be able to modify their program and progressively bring that person to a greater state of health and fitness.

Having said all this, what do we really want from our spines? The simple answer is, everything. The spine is the hanger from which we suspend the rest of our skeleton, the muscles, fat, and tissue that flesh us out, and the clothes that we wear to hide our nakedness and give us "style." The spine is the "rebar" that reinforces our structure within the foundation of feet, legs, and hips. Each vertebra is required to move independently yet also to work together with those above and below. In addition to this framework for the body to ride upon, the nerves running down the core of the spinal column communicate all the messages to and from the brain, limbs, vital organs, and sensory receptors of the body. We demand that it absorb constant vibration as we walk down the street, and bend, twist, and contort in all directions, while still protecting the central nerve core, the vital lifeline for our activity. It is no small task. It is obvious that the spine deserves every care we can give it to maintain both strength and flexibility. Enjoying the considerable range of motion of the human body requires constant maintenance.

Standing and walking are two of the most important things in human life. Proper walking, the more difficult of these two, depends on proper standing. In turn, in karate, without mastery of stance, walking, kicking and the forms are impossible to perform.

•

*Masutatsu Oyama
1923–94*

The effect of gravity also requires that we work on elongation of the entire spine with careful attention to maintaining the spacing between vertebrae. This relentless force can leave its stamp on the human body, and opposing muscles must be in good shape to avoid early aging or postural anomalies. When compressed over time, or suddenly in an accident, the disc material between vertebrae (a kind of cartilaginous jelly encased in a fibrous coating or shell) can bulge and push on nerves or vessels in the area. In more extreme cases, this casing can rupture and the interior jelly oozes out. This material is very irritating to surrounding tissue. These impingements can cause pain or numbness in other areas of the body, particularly down the legs, as well as nervous tension and sapping of energy. This is the condition referred to by the expression "slipped disc." In fact, the disc is not slipped at all, but as a mental image it is useful in visualizing the type of shearing action that can cause an injury. It occurs because one section of the spine is stiff and not moving fluidly between vertebrae as when the links in a bicycle chain seize and the pedal slips. The spine will often "give way" between these sections, and these trigger points can produce recurring problems.

The healthy spine is not, in fact, straight. Although it should be free of curves when viewed from the rear; if you were able to observe with x-ray vision from the side, you would see the lower lumbar and cervical spine curving inwards, and the thoracic outwards, from our imaginary straight line. What you have to feel when the "back is straight" then, is a spine free of tension or pain, with shoulders and pelvis slung freely within the framework. Every time you move, even to take a simple step, this architecture will change.

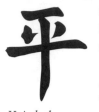

Hei: *balance, or peace*

The martial artist learns to find a center in all this structure, one in which energy flows freely and strength is at a maximum. Walking is, after all, merely a controlled fall, in which the forward-tilting body is repeatedly caught and supported by the right and left legs alternating in turn. Complex movement works from basic principles and constant unconscious adjustment of an internal gyroscope. The martial artist consciously trains this mechanism so that it can run on autopilot while he seeks to unbalance the system of his opponent. To do so, the martial artist wants upon a strong framework that will hold its form even when completely relaxed. He needs smooth mechanical workings where the muscles are not tensed, because he relies upon this relaxed state for sensitive reflexes and lightning fast speed. He also knows that to sustain vigorous activity over prolonged periods requires being able to rest muscle fiber between power states, even in quickly repeated actions.

Swing the Pendulum

Stance: In *fudo-dachi*, or "rooted stance," with feet two shoulder widths apart, and aligned at a 90° angle.

Action: Place hands on thighs and use them as sensors to feel the body weight shifting in the manner of a pendulum. Imagine the pendulum string fixed to the top of the head, holding the plumb, in this case the hips, free of tension, thus straightening the spine by the effect of gravity. Feel within the body as if you are sitting and floating in space without the need of any support under the buttocks. Keep knees gently flexed and slowly swing the hips forward and backward, with the head stationary. Let the muscles of the hip area, abdomen, and lower back achieve a point free of tension, with a gentle and enjoyable natural breathing pattern.

Duration: Play with the gravity. Instead of feeling it on the shoulders, head and spine, visualize the string pulling up to lighten the weight carried by the legs. Start with full oscillations and then decrease the amplitude until reaching a middle point where the pendulum can come to rest.

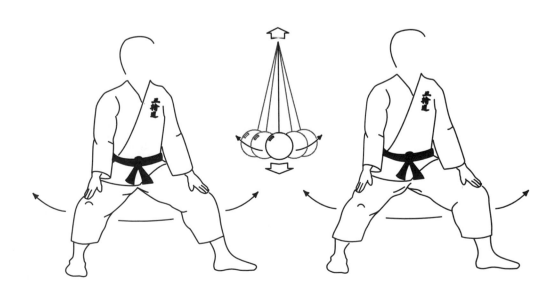

Mountain & River
Linked Series

Stance: With feet two shoulder widths apart, pivot both feet 90° to the right. Raise arms with hands together, reaching for the sky *(a)*. Legs should be straight but not locked.

Action: Bend the forward knee until the thigh is parallel to the floor, raising the rear heel, and keeping the spine vertical *(b)*. Hold for three breath cycles and concentrate on balance.

For the second phase, lift your hips and place the rear heel on the floor so that the foot is at a 45° angle with toes turned outward. Drop your hands to the sides of the forward foot and straighten both legs *(c)*, raising the hips but keeping the upper body bent forward, with chest close to forward knee. Hold and exhale for three breath cycles. Next, place both hands palm down on the floor to the left side of the forward foot *(d)*. Allow rear leg to extend behind you, raising the rear knee and heel and dropping the hips toward the floor. Feel the gentle stretch in the hip, groin, and upper thigh. Rest your weight on the whole forward foot, the ball of the rear foot and the hands. Hold and exhale for three breath cycles. For the last phase of the series, position the left knee and instep on the floor and gently sit on the rear heel *(e)*. With the front leg straight, bring the chest to the right thigh as deeply as you can but without forcing the stance. Hold for three breath cycles.

To return, raise the hips until the knees are at a 90° angle and the torso vertical, then put the left toes on the floor and return to the start position in a relaxed and gradual way.

Turn and repeat on the other side.

Level: Beginners may not be able to drop the hip enough in the first phase without losing balance. Remember, balance comes first, with flexibility and strength second. The same problem might occur with when straightening the leg in the second phase. Extend and straighten slowly until you feel the gentle tension.

Comments: Ensure that the rear knee is raised off the floor in *(b)* and *(d)*. Keep the spine straight, and do not bounce. Take care not to stand up too quickly. Let the phases of this exercise flow smoothly together.

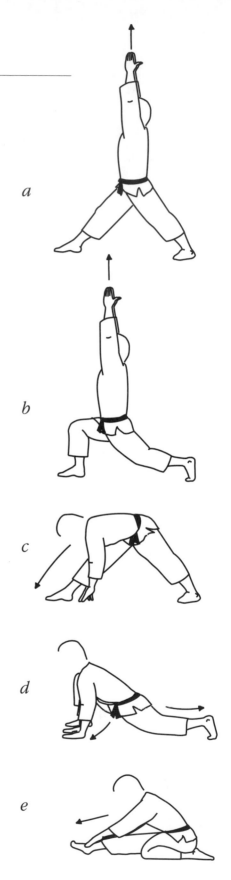

a

b

c

d

e

Full Extension

Stance: Lie on your back, with legs straight and together, with arms fully extended above head.

Action: Extend toes and fingers, reaching and stretching with hands side by side as far as possible above head. Tense and hold for a count of three, then relax and exhale.

Duration: Repeat three times.

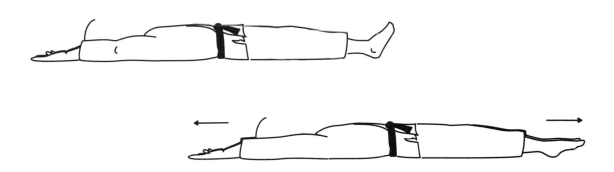

Cat Stretch

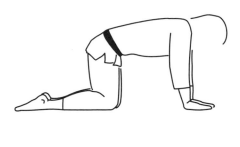

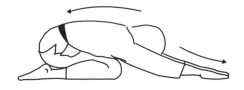

Stance: From a *seiza*, kneeling position, sit on the heels with the torso vertical.

Action: Bend forward with arms extended in front of you until hands touch the floor. Begin with hands directly under shoulders and knees under hips. Keeping spine and head straight, arms extended, slowly sit back on the heels, feeling the elongation of the spine. Exhale as you bend.

Duration: Maintain the crouch for four breathing cycles.

Secrets of the Martial Arts

- In order to move well, the martial artist requires a body that is well tuned and in good running order, one in which reflexes, balance, strength, flexibility, and intrinsic energy are responding in harmony. This is not possible without good alignment of the spine.

- Keeping the upper body erect and the spine in line permits quick, balanced movement and the application of centrifugal force, using the extended limbs as striking, blocking, and deflecting weapons.

- Although the *seiza* position (with head and spine in line) requires some practice and flexibility to achieve correct alignment, its usefulness in locating the breathing and center of gravity around the *hara* is important.

- Many of the martial arts breathing exercises, when properly performed, actually bring the spine into good alignment and reduce the compression of the vertebrae.

- The success of the martial artist, in terms of being able to train without injury and perform increasingly demanding technique, depends on being attentive and dedicated to good form.

- The martial artist works hard on the conditioning of the body, not just to be able to perform actively, but also for the reward of relaxing without strain, tension, or weakness.

- Bodybuilding, and spot exercises that focus only on attractive muscular appearance can interfere with flexibility and be a source of repetitive stress injury.

- Martial arts training can be recommended as an exercise program because of its supervised, progressive approach, emphasizing good technique and correct body position.

- Patience, discipline, and an ability to maintain focus in the present moment assist greatly in achieving the benefits of the martial arts exercise regimen.

- It is obvious that the spine deserves every care we can give it to maintain both strength and flexibility. Enjoying the considerable range of motion of the human body requires constant maintenance.

Chapter 4

Flexible Body, Flexible Mind

THE martial artist begins learning technique from the first bow at the doorway of the *dojo* (literally, "a place to study the Way"). Fingers and feet together, eyes ahead, back straight, left foot moving, arms crossing, he or she engages in endless correction of form and feeling. Technique is polished, cardiovascular performance is improved, muscles are strengthened, speed is increased, reflexes are sharpened, and yes, eventually comes the ability to do jumping, spinning kicks. With good instruction a martial artist will learn early in his practice that all this effort shares the common goal of flexibility—uniting the desire for strength with the ability to yield, both mentally and physically.

By surrendering to the idea that every step and every breath, forward and backward, in and out, is part of the whole process, and by examining, exploring, and trying new ways, we are "doing" martial arts. This can perhaps be easiest to understand for the white belt "beginner," who doesn't know anything else, and hardest for the black belt "expert," who is afraid to find out what else he doesn't know.

Some of the basic principles can be the most difficult to grasp and accept. Learning, for example, that the ability to stretch is not flexibility, relaxed is not flaccid or weak, strong is not always hard, effort is not always rewarded, and that a mistake is something for which to be grateful, can be difficult for even the most experienced student of martial arts. Although these conundrums will be revisited at every stage of the training, the sooner we truly understand the nature of these questions, the less important their answers will seem. As problems become less pressing, often the solutions begin to flow naturally. Martial arts are about big things and small things, gross motor movements and the merest wink of a flexor. Satisfaction rather than gratification must be the goal of the student, who will take many small steps before being able to map progress with landmarks.

One of the most valuable concepts of Eastern instructional philosophy is crystallized in the Japanese word *nyuanshin*. Commonly translated "beginner's mind," it refers to an attitude that is receptive and open to learning, one that anticipates and accepts what is being taught throughout the entire course of training. "Receptive mind," might be a definition clearer than the literal "beginner's mind," because, as most teachers will attest, new students often have preconceptions that need to be dispelled before learning can begin.

It is very natural for us to file new information into our previously established categories rather than revising our way of looking at things and what we think they mean. Although occasionally we are asked to abandon what we previously held to be true, the principle of *nyuanshin* does not ask the student of martial arts to relinquish judgment, deductive reasoning, or even intuitive insight. Quite the contrary, it demands that the martial artist bring all these faculties to bear on the problem of learning about a complex physical system, while operating within the context of a mental and spiritual awakening. It can be challenging for the teacher to answer the questions of beginners fully when they have yet to develop a working "vocabulary" of principles. Sometimes students just have to accept, for the moment at least, that things are just the way the teacher says. By embracing and "just doing," understanding will often occur. The Zen underpinnings of martial arts poses these learning situations as philosophical dilemmas, which have been expressed historically in storytelling and myth.

Students of martial arts cannot, however, subsume themselves completely to the Way of even the best teachers, for ultimately they still must "own" the experience, do the learning, and walk the path (albeit one well trodden by those who have gone before). Hopefully, they will encounter something unique along their own way. One of the ways in which the traditional learning system benefits the martial arts, is the development of the student as a teacher. A successful school, or *ryu*, is one in which the fundamental principles and practices can be passed on by the senior students. In the process of teaching, advanced practitioners have the opportunity to examine their understanding of the basics at their own level. Working with partners and helping with beginners is an important part of the training, and is the reason for the formal respect and titles accorded more senior students.

The preparation of the body must also be undertaken with patience, remembering that the body has a beginner's mind too. Its tissues and systems must learn and become accustomed to changes in conditioning. "Muscle memory" is acquired after some practice, and the rate of learning is different from one individual to another. Coordination is often difficult at the early stages, but comes eventually, and even advanced students will sometimes confuse individual elements of combinations. After a period of inactivity or injury, caution must be exercised to retrain or refresh the body and assist its re-integration with the mind.

The martial artist needs to be keenly aware of his physical and mental mechanisms and how they are responding. He should be willing to change and improve, even when he thinks a skill has been acquired. It can be much more difficult to correct even a subtle error later, when it has become ingrained. This is another reason for the strong emphasis on continuous, repetitive practice of basics. The student hopes to achieve a dynamic where constant conscious correction is not required, but where there still exists an automatic unconscious feedback. A martial artist wants an autopilot that is alert to change. Achieving this requires that part of *nyuanshin* that is rooted in patience, diligence, and forgiveness for being a beginner. It is always hard to embrace one's own errors, but this is the only way to learn. By extension, martial artists who receive good instruction will also learn to forgive the errors of their fellow students (and even their teachers) and help them along the Way.

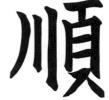

Jun:
*gentleness,
or ease*

Martial arts training systematically takes students through steps to educate the body in fitness and technique, and more importantly, should provide them with the tools to evaluate progress in their own development, thereby making it easier to acquire new skills in the future. Advanced students will look forward to learning something new, and not be overly concerned with the mistakes that will be made as part of that learning process.

In a good school, beginners are honored by this allowance for error. Progress that may seem small, when compared with the long path senior students have followed, is nevertheless recognized and applauded. Good attitude and effort are rewarded by consistent improvement without injury. The secret is to pay attention to the instruction, and practice, practice, practice.

Learning to be relaxed, both physically and mentally, is an essential part of the training, and comes from being relaxed about learning. Accordingly, most martial artists find that they make breakthroughs in other areas of their lives, such as jobs or hobbies, where they come to look at things in new ways, or they attempt courses or projects that previously seemed intimidating. As their body strengthens, reflexes quicken, and confidence grows, other sports and activities become open to them. For older students who were never considered athletic in traditional areas, the recognition that they *can* in fact learn to be skilled athletes, is very exciting and life changing. Overcoming performance fears can make skills such as public speaking seem possible even to those previously paralyzed by such experiences.

A martial art is a discipline that stresses excellence. This pursuit, however, is one that is acquired through dedication and is not necessarily one that comes naturally. As in many areas of study, those who do very well in the beginning stages and take to the training without much effort often become bogged down as intermediate or advanced students, when they reach plateaus at which progress has apparently slowed. It is then that the "tortoises" of the group, who simply plod along trying to get better, are able to stick with the training and not allow frustration to spoil their enjoyment of the activity.

Martial arts schools that have competition as a major goal may sometimes discourage participants who are able to achieve excellence without proving themselves better than their fellow students. This is unfortunate, for such students can prove a valuable asset. By working with their classmates rather than trying to outdo them, the learning environment improves, cooperation flourishes, and a spirit of camaraderie pervades the class. While martial arts training might well enhance qualities that elite competitors need to have, it does not necessarily follow that the pressures of tournaments, and the negative attitudes sometimes accompanying them, convey benefits to those sincerely traveling the Way.

The martial arts *dojo* is a special environment designed to encourage a sensible and safe approach to the study of ideas and techniques that could be dangerous if applied incorrectly or for the wrong reasons. A real *dojo* functions properly because of correct and safe teaching, and traditions and etiquette of behavior that favor learning, concentration, and commitment. The *dojo* is not a special place by itself, but becomes special because of the attitude and training of the people in it. It does not have to be fancy, particularly well equipped, or severely austere. A *dojo* can be created anywhere that someone makes a conscious decision to train in a certain way.

How do we use this mental and spiritual framework of learning and thinking to achieve very physical tasks? By shaping the physical goals of the body, such as strength and flexibility, around the philosophical principles, an interesting sharing of metaphors takes place. "Going with the flow" describes a body moving in space as a physical reality, while at the same time its prescription for mental adjustment is no less real.

A good workout has its own structure too. A training session always begins with a good warm-up. This is an opportunity for the conscious and unconscious mental processes to connect with and move into syn-chronization with the body. Moving the mind away from the distractions of the day to focus on the present moment is necessary to coordinate the reflexes and responses of physical movement.

The warm-up begins with exercises that gently loosen the muscles and joints and gradually proceeds to larger movements that raise the body temperature slightly. As the tissues become warmer, some light stretching and rotation of the limbs can be performed. Although martial artists are known for their ability to stretch, they are care-ful to attempt this type of activity only when the limbs are adequately prepared. Exercises to increase flexibility and intense stretching are ideally done toward the end of a training session in a very warm state, but before fatigue has taken over.

After a standard warm-up, the body and mind are ready for more vigorous and demanding training. Even so, as new exercises are introduced, the student will first exe-cute the technique slowly a few times, building up to full power only when sure it is being executed properly. This protects the body and the training partner from damage. In periods of intense practice, it is up to the mind to stay focused and relaxed to maintain the body "in the groove" and to guard against loss of control. As fatigue sets in, this mental vigilance becomes even more vital, and is in fact what martial artists are practicing when they take simple techniques and perform them at full intensity. By concentrating on correct form and abdominal breathing rather than the effects of fatigue, one's physical limits can be stretched and mental signals rearranged.

This is when the martial artist tries to remember the relaxed mental state that is practiced in *seiza*. Once the muscle memory can take over the mechanics of a tech-nique, the mind is free to adjust naturally to changes in the moment, to calm the breathing, and to find a measure of stillness amidst the noise and movement. This is not something that comes magically or automatically from the meditation sessions alone, but must be practiced with the body. Sometimes it helps to imagine the responses of the mind as a radio that must be tuned to a clear frequency, and readjusted when it drifts off the station.

Part of this attitude involves taking a pro-active rather than a re-ac-tive approach to life and training. On both a macro and a micro scale,

One of the most striking features of karate *is that it may be engaged in by anybody, young or old, strong or weak, male or female. Further, one need not even have an opponent for practice purposes. Nor is there any need for a specially made uniform. Even a* dojo *is unnecessary: a person can practice* karate *in his own yard. Of course, anyone truly determined to master the various* kata *must do so at a proper* dojo, *but someone whose desire is merely to stay healthy and to train his mind and spirit may do so by practicing* karate *by himself.*

•

Gichin Funakoshi
1868–1957

martial arts teaches us to step inside and act, rather than wait to be acted upon. While this concept has to be interpreted carefully when clarifying what self-defense is, it is helpful in illustrating everything from the dynamics of a technique to the internal spiritual energy that must be summoned when fatigued or frightened.

In a more everyday sense, a useful visualization for training or running or even walking in a crowded shopping mall, is that of stepping on a ball or globe that you turn with your feet as you move. By actively engaging the sphere with your energy, strength, and balance, rather than being controlled by the movement, a subtle but important shift in attitude takes place. By learning to tune to this channel, many physiological and social obstacles can be eventually overcome. Another useful visualisation might be that of running on uneven ground in the woods, feeling the feet landing and pushing off, seeking out the next hold on the surface that allows you to spin the sphere. Your hands reach out to move branches or lean against the smooth bark of a tree, to balance the gyroscope that keeps the ride fluid, calm, and smooth at the center.

Acquiring all of these skills and benefits requires that one approach martial arts training with intelligence. It is ironic that at the same time that martial arts have mass appeal due to the exploitation of brainless cultural stereotypes they are equally popular among professional athletes and coaches, not necessarily for physical conditioning, but for their mental benefits. The true philosophy and spirituality of martial arts are in fact very much at odds with the violent contests and humorous slapstick portrayed by the popular media.

The feats of skill and endurance that have become the hallmarks of the martial arts are by and large the result of training and utilizing the resources of the body intelligently. Recognizing the structural physics of the human body, and bringing its kinetic and chemical resources to bear, accounts for most of the training spectrum. When their philosophical and spiritual elements are in play, the martial arts become very powerful forces indeed. By choosing to wield the body in the manner of a controlled snap of a whip, rather than the awkward swing of a piece of lumber, different outcomes will result.

Flexibility in martial art begins in the mind, is led by the will, and nurtured by the breathing. As a famous jazz musician once wrote, "it don't mean a thing if it ain't got that swing." As training progresses, the body gets stronger and the technique more accurate, but all is for naught if self-awareness and character development have not occurred as well.

Being able to do the "splits" is a common obsession of beginners in martial arts training. Movies and posters have exaggerated the value of this ability, and although many techniques require the stretching of certain muscles to achieve a full range of motion, it is really not that

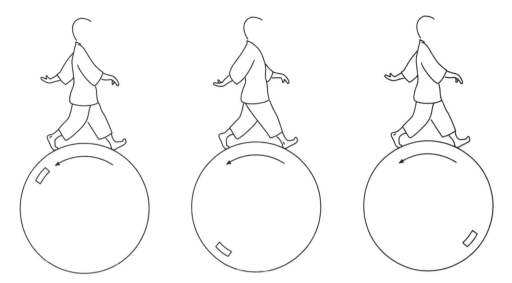

You can alter your mental relationship with your environment
by visualizing that you are moving the earth under your feet.

important compared with the need for fluidity and responsiveness that true flexibility provides. It is important to recognize that stretching muscle fiber, such as when performing the splits, is not necessarily improving flexibility, and in fact overstretching some areas can impede the mobility of joints by causing stiffness or irritation of muscle tissue, tendons, and ligaments.

A common error made by those attempting to touch the floor when standing, for example, or trying to generally reach new lengths in a stretch, is a bouncing action referred to as ballistic stretching. While in certain situations this can be useful exercise for the fully conditioned body, (for example, to strengthen flexors), it is inappropriate for a warm-up and can be damaging to the muscle fiber. In the process of bouncing one can have the illusion of improving stretching range, but the fibers have a tendency to shorten and stiffen with a contracting reflex, and for the beginner this can cause soreness or pain, and reduced stretch after cooling-down. This type of exercise, or stretching without a proper warm-up, can damage the tendons, where they connect to the muscles or to the bone, and can produce an injury that takes a long time to heal. This can also place undue strain on the ligaments that are working to maintain the stability of joints. Good martial arts teachers will emphasize gradual but consistent development of strength and flexibility, and will discourage the inclination to show off or overreach; their students will be rewarded with a painless transformation of the structural tensions in the body's architecture.

It is rarely necessary for the purposes of self-defense to be able to kick over the opponent's head or contort the body into unusual positions. However, the ability to do so as a conditioning exercise when fully warmed up should allow for a higher degree of flexibility in the "cold" state. There is a joke in the martial arts about the practitioner who, when confronted by a mugger, asks him to wait while he warms up, so that he can demonstrate some fancy technique to disarm him. This cautionary tale acknowledges that one can rarely choose the time or place when the body will be called upon to perform, and that it is more important to achieve a functional state of balanced readiness, than the occasional extreme state of high performance.

The martial artist cultivates a mental image of flexibility that is not just loose, soft, or malleable, but incorporates a tensile strength that prevents overstretching, slippage, and fatigue failure. Traditional masters often invoked the example of a living tree, usually a willow or a pine, to illustrate the appropiate combination of properties. Their heavily snow-laden branches are able to yield without breaking, while even rigid planks of wood milled from their trunk can be steamed into graceful structural curves.

Flexibility has to be understood as an improved arrangement of the body segments that allows for fluid mobility without strain. Stretching generally involves one muscle or muscle group, and as an "ability" is something that can be shown or demonstrated, but not necessarily used. One might easily argue that the time involved in improving one's stretch might be better spent on exercises to improve technique, breathing, and overall flexibility.

Those who do not have profound stretching ability can still perform well by coordinating all the elements that make up good technique. In a high kick for example, stretching is only one factor involved in an efficient and powerful delivery that has good reach. Equally important are foot position, arch of the back, neck and head position, direction and focus of the eyes, relaxation of shoulders and hips, position of hands in the guard, and exhalation of the breath. Clearly, if the goal of the martial artist is a technique that works, not just one that shows well for a photo or a tournament judge, more practice of technique is required than of stretching.

There are many misconceptions about flexibility. As we have mentioned, many newcomers to a martial art school will state as one of their goals that they would like to improve their "stretch," specifically be able to do the splits, because they think it looks impressive and will be expected of them for black belt. Unfortunately, many people never venture near a *dojo* because they believe they will be unable to perform such a feat, or worse, have heard of torture-like devices and exercises that will be forced upon them. Many will claim that they are too old to learn such movements. Those brave enough to venture to the registration desk, when asked about any medical condition that could affect their training, will reply that: "I'm not very flexible. I can't touch my toes or do the splits," as if it were an illness or injury that limits them.

A good martial arts teacher will insure that his students seek improvement in their flexibility as a result of consistent regular practice, good warm-ups and cool-downs, and stretching that is longer and deeper by gradual degrees. It is more important to maintain flexibility on a daily basis and stretch intensively only occasionally. One should stretch only when the muscles are fully warm and to the extent appropriate for the level of activity performed that day. It is prudent to know your limits and wisely improve upon them. A good stretching exercise will create a sensation of sweet discomfort, not pain, and there should be a feeling of release in tension from the other areas of the body not directly involved in the stretch. It helps to smile, relax the face, jaw, and tongue, and wriggle the toes to ensure that you are not overtense or causing damage. Exhalation while stretching is vital. Good breathing practice before and after a session of stretching will help the circulation of oxygen and removal of waste by-products from the tissues by the bloodstream.

True flexibility is not measured by the degree of final stretch in an exercise, but is more effectively measured by where you start the next time. Even so, abilities from day to day will be affected by how intense the last class was (was there some new exercise?), outside activities (the Saturday softball game or the office picnic), your work-day footwear (high heels or construction boots), sleeping position, etc. Factors

Structure, physics, and mechanics of movement will
affect the effort required for any task or technique.

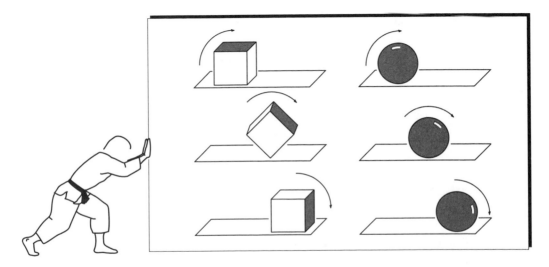

such as the weather, humidity, room temperature, and even what you ate for breakfast can also enter into the picture.

Progress in this area is relative and individual. Comparing the height of your kick or the arch of your spine to someone who began at a higher level but did not improve as much, is counterproductive. Here the mental flexibility of patience and taking satisfaction in personal progress will play a more important role than daily stretching. Dedication of some extra time to flexibility will show results. Remember that many people who seem very flexible are naturally so because of an abnormality of collagen in their joints and ligaments. Contortionists who we see in exhibitions are generally "blessed" with this condition. Unfortunately, it is difficult for these people to participate in some activities because it is too easy for them to dislocate joints or break bones under resistance. Those who are overly mobile in their joints have to exercise caution in martial arts by strengthening the muscles around the joints and consciously constraining techniques to avoid hyperextension. It can be harder for them to achieve flexibility and resilience because their joints, ligaments, and tendons are "opening" when they do the exercise, rather than the muscle fibers in the target zone stretching. Caution must also be exercised by the martial artist with a yoga background, because some of the exercises such as the full-lotus position (the cross-legged sitting often used for meditation) can over-stretch ligaments in the knee. This has the potential to cause instability when kicking or standing in martial arts exercises.

It is true that some martial arts styles, such as some of the schools of *karate*, place great importance on the hard, lean body and even go so far as to prescribe the toughening of hands, shins, and feet to give or receive blows with hard objects. Most, however, recognize the need for a relaxed or untensed state between techniques to maximize speed from one movement to the next. At the other end of the spectrum, *aikido* avoids the blunt meeting of force with force and emphasizes yielding, deflection, and redirection of an attack. Yet, no one who has undertaken the numerous falls, rolls, and rising from the ground of

B EGINNER . . . is not aware of his mistakes while others notice them easily.

I NTERMEDIATE . . . is aware of mistakes to correct and others can see the corrections.

A DVANCED . . . is aware of mistakes that others do not see and when corrected only the teacher notices.

T EACHER . . . is aware of mistakes unseen by others and makes corrections known only to himself.

M ASTER . . . knows that he still makes mistakes and strives to perfect them even though he knows perfection is impossible.

even a basic training class would ever question the strength and resiliency required in the body of the *aikido* practitioner.

This concept of soft and hard in the martial arts can be difficult to understand, especially for those who come to the training already physically strong, and those who have been unduly influenced by demonstrations of board-breaking or media portrayals of martial artists with superhuman strength. Relying on strength alone to resist an assault can lead to defeat when you are facing someone bigger and stronger, or when you are injured, sick, or aged, or simply when your opponent knows how to use your own force against you. It is this way that martial arts can teach the diminutive person to use intelligence, breathing, speed, relaxation, timing, and knowledge of balance and technique to overcome the stronger attacker.

Martial arts training is a very tactile experience. From self-awareness of one's own body comes knowledge of an opponent's body. Practicing with various partners develops the ability to judge resistance and flexibility of limbs and joints. Knowing the pain thresholds and breaking points comes from close and careful work on grappling and choking techniques. This training requires trust and sensitivity, and is one of the most demanding and rewarding aspects of good practice and good teaching.

While most people understand that martial arts training creates a physical body that can be used as a tool to perform tasks, what is less well known is the extent to which executing the tasks becomes a tool for the development of the body and psyche. We have discussed how a relaxed mind state can assist the body in achieving its objectives, but it is equally important to observe how the physical state can produce effects in the mental and spiritual dimension. The physical act of willing the muscles to "imitate" a different emotional state can often produce the feelings that accompany that attitude, thus releasing constraint or uplifting the spirit. Similar effects can be observed with respect to breathing, body alignment, and general vigorous activity. In self-defense, presenting an image that is confident and relaxed will assist the mind in staying prepared and discourage those who prey upon weakness. The vital ability to control which muscles are tensed, and when, allows the martial artist to influence both his physical and mental states.

Most martial artists practice in bare feet or in light footwear that still permits good contact with the ground. The stimulation of nerve endings and the massage effect of the feet in direct contact with various surfaces is extremely beneficial. The feet and ankles contain many small bones, ligaments, tendons, and muscles that need exercise and conditioning in the same way as other areas of the body. With attention to good warm-up and correct foot position in stances, many students find that weakness in arches and other related foot ailments diminish, and in some cases disappear with the training. Strengthening of the muscles provides natural arch support, better weight distribution, and improved mechanics within the foot.

This is like Mount Fuji's being concealed by a single tree thick with branches and leaves, and my not being able to see it. But how can Mount Fuji be concealed by a single tree? It is simply because of the narrowness of my vision and because the tree stands in the way of my vision that Mount Fuji cannot be seen. We go on thinking that the tree is concealing Mount Fuji. Yet it is due to the narrowness of my vision.

•

Takuan Soho

1573–1645

In some martial arts, various parts of the foot are brought into contact with practice pads or the opponent's anatomy, and many different foot positions may be used in stances and kicking. To form these correctly requires strength and flexibility in the joints greater than that required by walking or running. Modern athletic shoes, which provide support, allow the foot and ankle to be "lazy." Training the foot to provide the foundation for good technique, improves the muscular and skeletal balance in the rest of the body through the legs, hips and back, and is an often overlooked way of improving spinal alignment. This effect is similar to that obtained by orthotic devices that are placed in shoes, but instead reduces the need for such devices.

The physical exercises of martial arts training act as self-massage on the body itself. Sustained abdominal breathing massages the inner organs, including the intestines. The lymphatic system circulates more readily when pumped by muscular contraction (and respiratory efficiency), which aids in the function of the immune system. Grappling techniques massage the hands, wrists, forearms, and when performed correctly, gently loosen the joints and stretch the muscles. The hands are constantly opening and closing, grabbing and releasing. Ground grappling massages the buttocks, back, shoulders, and neck, and the repetitive rolling, falling, and rising to the standing position have similar effects that are both relaxing and strengthening.

Bilateral motion of the body is strongly emphasized in martial arts training. The student is discouraged from favoring his dominant side, so that equal proficiency in skills on both the left and right sides is developed. Extra attention is devoted to the weaker side, with more repetitions, resistance, or time spent working that side. Although it is best to learn a technique on the more proficient side, when practicing one should begin and end on the other, weaker side. This is important not only to avoid displaying a weakness to an opponent, but also to maintain a balance in the strength of muscles across the pelvis, back, and shoulders that help control the alignment of the spine. We may appear to be straight on the frontal plane, and have natural curves on the lateral, but a top view might indicate a twist in the relaxed position of the pelvis or shoulders. This can inhibit flexibility, or lead to a shearing effect of the vertebrae under a load or unusual stress.

Bilateral motion is also incorporated in many techniques. Pushing and pulling or pressing and lifting with opposite hands occurs frequently, and although these motions may be required for leverage or locking, the benefit, from a repetitive training point of view, is the balancing of strength in the limbs across the spine. Other examples are found in techniques involving an action-reaction sequence, such as an elbow striking backward as a punch is thrust forward, or a hand and arm extending out to one side when a high side kick is performed in the opposite direction.

As explained here and there, the gist of judo *rests on pliable action of mind and body. The word "pliable," however, never means weakness: something like free broad-mindedness or adaptability which is akin to the true meaning. The gist of* judo *is to find the original characteristic of the man in the ever-growing nature and to personify true freedom of thought or action.*

•

Kyuzo Mifune
1883–1965

There is a good deal of torsion dynamic in the execution of martial arts techniques. The secret to the strength and power able to be delivered, and the speed in which blows can be avoided, lies in the turning movement of the hips. This motion is similar to the leading from the hips of the golf swing or the tennis backhand, but is used in almost every move, both subtle and obvious. This is why it is so important that the hips, pelvis, and lower back be free to move, and also be strong, flexible, and balanced in their supporting musculature. It is also vital that the shoulders be down and relaxed and the fists held gently until the moment of impact, so that the hip motion is uninhibited and fluid. Beginners with developed upper-body strength can find it difficult to even locate their hip strength when punching. It is even harder for them to use it effectively, because they find it natural to exert their power with upper arms and shoulders alone. If these muscles are flexed they can impart a tightness to the chest and back that doesn't allow the hips to move. Teaching tools to correct this and illustrate to the student what is happening include hypertensing the upper body by raising the shoulders, clenching the fists and face, and then letting go. By trying to twist the hips gently in each of these positions, the student begins to see the limitations he may be placing on his own movement. Crossing the arms over the chest, with the forearms in the opposite sleeve of the *gi* (practice uniform), can allow walking, kicking, or moving from one stance to the next take place without upper body tension, thereby freeing the pelvis to tilt and the hips to rotate. Demonstrating the difference in grip strength (by grabbing your own knees in a sitting position for example), with the shoulders raised and then the shoulders lowered and relaxed, can illustrate clearly the effect of body physics, breathing, and center of gravity to the student who believes that strength is all.

Psychiatrists have noted that breaking mental patterns, many of which relate to specific body language, can release tension and bottled up emotions and allow for new ideas, ways of coping, and reinterpretation of events. Similar results occur when physical patterns change or limitations are overcome in the martial arts. As we age, we become accustomed to certain ways of doing things, and our ideas about ourselves and what we can do become fixed. Many of these assumptions are challenged through the course of martial arts training.

A simple example will illustrate how what we feel is natural is often simply what has become usual. Most of us fold our arms across our chest or clap our hands one way only. Left over right, or right over left. Changing that pattern requires no significant effort or skill, but can require much practice. One feels right and the other not, and often the beginner will say "but I can't do it that way." It is not that they don't know how, or lack the ability to learn, but they just feel unaccustomed to the sensation, especially compared to the old way. Many advanced students are also faced with this challenge when correcting old errors or attempting alternative approaches, especially with a new teacher. Many teachers will confirm that it is often easier to teach an absolute beginner to achieve an intermediate level, than a person with previous experience or advanced skills in another style or approach. It can be frustrating to unlearn and relearn, especially if the muscle and reflex responses are similar. It is on these occasions that the principle of the beginner's mind must be invoked.

When the body-mind state has been sufficiently conditioned that it can operate in balance when placed under pressure, the rewards and benefits of an intense workout at an advanced level increase exponentially. This high degree of training can allow for leaps in understanding, and realizations that can have significant impact on the individual. Functioning well at this level can also produce a higher order of relaxation, both within and after the training session. This is not to be confused with exhaustion and, in fact, one of the signs of having achieved this experience is that, after a short recovery period, you feel like your battery is charged with new energy rather than drained. This will, of course, depend on the rhythm of the class and the experience of the practitioner. It is also true that many beginners have a similar reaction in their first weeks of classes, because they feel energized and excited by the workout and this new world that they have entered. This keenness to "do another class" has to be tempered by the instructor or senior students, because the beginner's body is simply not ready to sustain numerous classes in a row without healthy rest in between. As well, for both beginner and advanced students, the intense euphoria induced by endorphins, efficient respiration, and the satisfaction that comes from moving well, can interfere with the focus and control necessary for good, safe practice.

The goal of the training martial artist must be to achieve excellence rather than perfection. Perfect practice makes excellence possible, and although seemingly perfect moments are attained by those on this quest, they are rarely duplicated or sustained for long. These fleeting "brushes with greatness" should stimulate the training rather than disappoint the perfectionist. The bad news is that there is no perfection in the martial arts, for they are grounded on the principle that there is always room for improvement. The good news is that with perseverance and an eye fixed on excellence, the Way is enjoyable, healthy, and rewarding—physically, mentally, and spiritually.

Martial arts teaches several lessons: Embrace your body as it is today. Work with it, and in it, so that it will be better tomorrow. Accept your mistakes and be happy when you recognize them, for it is only then that they can be corrected. Laugh when you fall down, and then get up and do it better next time. Respect the feedback of your teachers, because they have even more to teach you. As you exercise patience in yourself, so must they.

> B EGINNER . . . one who is looking for more answers.
>
> A DVANCED . . . one who is looking for more questions.

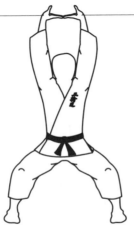

Abdominals

Stance: Lie on back, legs flexed with the feet on the ground, hands raised forward in front. Keep the chin one fist distance away from the chest, and look to the knees.

Action: Slowly contract the abdomen and raise the upper back from the floor, reaching for the knees. Exhale, returning slowly and gently to the floor.

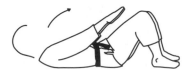

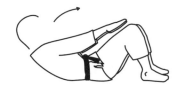

Duration: Do two sets of ten repetitions.

Comments: The degree of effort will change when the hands reach above the knees. Focus on your abdominal muscles only and do not raise your torso completely. Rest between sets with the back on the floor and breathe comfortably. This is not a flexibility exercise but a way to build abdominal strength to avoid back problems. We recommend attention and caution and not doing them when tired.

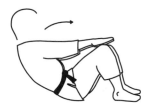

Hip Rotation

Stance: Stand with feet shoulder width apart.

Action: With hands on hips, gently rotate hips in a circular motion, beginning with small circles and spiralling outward. Make ten circles in each direction.

Comments: Allow knees and ankles to flex with the rotation. Maintain head at rest in the center position, moving body around it. Exhale.

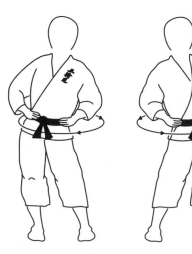

Front Knee Up

Stance: Stand with feet together. Balancing on the left foot, slowly raise the right knee while maintaining a straight spine. Grasp the shin with both hands.

Action: Exhale and bring the knee gently upward and in toward your abdomen, keeping the supporting leg straight and hips on a horizontal line.

Duration: Hold for a count of ten, then relax the position. Repeat on the other side.

Comments: Change legs in a slow and controlled fashion. When returning to the support of two feet, be very conscious of the body weight distribution and spinal alignment. If you find difficulty balancing, do the exercise in a corner or with a wall behind you. Work to control tilting by relaxing and exhaling slowly. Looking forward toward a distant point will help you, as well as maintaining a gentle tension on the abdominal muscles to tilt the pelvis upward. If necessary, bend the support knee slightly to drop the center of gravity. Keep the head and spine straight all the time as if they were pulled up by a string from the top of the head.

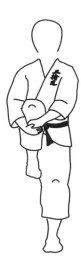

Raise Foot Backward

Stance: Start by balancing on left foot. Flex the right knee slowly, raising the foot behind you. Grasp the foot with one or both hands. Maintain a straight spine with hips horizontal.

Action: Exhale and bring the foot in close to the buttock, feeling a gentle stretch on the thigh and instep. Drop the shoulders and pull them backward in a open chest action.

Duration: Hold for a count of ten, then relax the position. Repeat on the other side.

Comments: Change legs, in a slow and controlled manner. Maintain balance by exhaling, relaxing, and tilting the pelvis upwards slightly.

Avoid letting the hip slip out of line to the side. Keep the flexed knee down and close to the base knee.

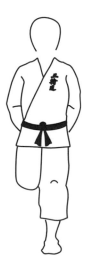
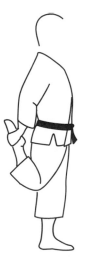

Hamstring Elongation, Center

Stance: Begin with feet two shoulder widths apart.

Action: Gradually lower upper body toward the floor, supporting your weight with the hands resting on the legs above the knees. Keeping spine and head in line, reach down with your hands in the center until you feel a gentle tension in the back of your legs.

Duration: Exhale, relax, and hold for a count of 20. Return slowly to the standing position, curling the spine up in a rolling motion that allows the head to rise last.

Level: It is not necessary for beginners to reach the floor. Continue to support the weight on the knees. If this exercise is done with proper technique, your flexibility will improve gradually.

Resist spreading your feet further apart or leaning forward in order to touch the floor. By doing so you are shifting the stretch to other muscles and cheating yourself out of the chance to improve.

For advanced elongation, allow the hands to slide down the legs and come together in the center. Reach gently.

Comments: Do not bounce, and do not stretch to the point of discomfort or pain. Keep the knee joint unlocked and take care not to hyperextend it.

Remember to exhale as you bend down and breathe normally in the hold position. Inhale as you return to the standing position. Keep eyes open, looking down and slightly forward. Avoid bending neck out of line.

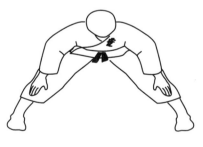

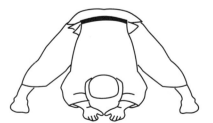

Hamstring Elongation, Individual Leg

Stance: Stand with feet two shoulder widths apart.

Action: Turn the upper body and head to a 45° angle and gradually lower the upper body, with chest moving toward the knee to the point of a relaxed stretch, allowing the hands to support the weight along the leg. Reach will vary according to state of warm-up or cool-down. Be careful to not overstretch. Keep head in line with spine, and do not bow or twist.

Duration: Exhale, relax, and hold for a count of 20. Return gently to the starting position and repeat on other side.

Level: If this exercise is done properly, your flexibility will improve gradually. For advanced elongation grab lower on the ankle.

Comments: Do not bounce and not stretch to the point of discomfort or pain. Keep the knee joint unlocked and take care to not hyperextend it.

Maintain spine and head position; lower chest to knee, not the head to knee. If proper position is not maintained the muscles of the back will be stretching and not the hamstrings. Remember to breathe normally in the hold position. Avoid twisting and pulling on the leg.

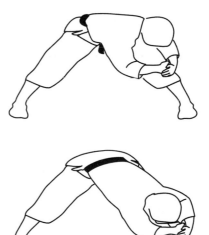

Achilles and Adductor Stretch

Stance: Stand with feet two shoulder widths apart.

Action: Bending forward slightly at the waist, support hands on upper thighs. Shift weight to one side as you gently begin to slide the other foot outward a few inches, maintaining the feet parallel to each other and soles flat on the floor. Keeping the heel of the supporting foot fully on the floor and the bent knee directly above that foot (pushing out gently with your elbow), continue to lower the body weight until you feel a gentle stretch in the inner thigh and the back of the ankle.

You may need to touch the floor in front of you or reach forward with both hands to maintain balance.

Duration: Hold for a count of 20. Rise slowly by placing hands on floor and shifting weight back to center and up. Repeat on the other side.

Level: It is more important to achieve the appropriate stretch than to lower yourself to the floor. Do not cheat by raising the heel of the supporting foot.

Comments: Keep both feet parallel and flat on the floor. Exercise caution with the position of the knees. Do not press down on the knee of the extended leg. Lower yourself slowly to maintain balance.

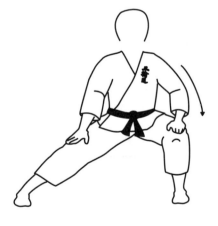

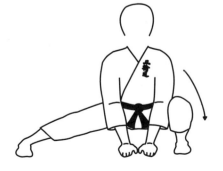

Hip Drop Stretch

Stance: Stand with feet two shoulder widths apart, pivot both feet to the left side, and drop right knee slowly to the floor.

Action: Place both hands palm down on the floor to the right side of the forward foot. Allow the rear leg to extend behind you, raising the rear knee and heel and dropping the hips toward the floor. Feel the gentle stretch in the hip, groin, and upper thigh. Hold and exhale for a count of 20, resting your weight on the whole of the forward foot, the ball of the rear foot, and the hands.

For the second phase, lift the hips and place the rear heel on the floor so the foot is at a 45° angle with toes toward the outside. Shift hands to each side of the forward foot and straighten both legs, raising the hips but keeping the upper body bent forward, with chest close to forward knee. Hold and exhale for a count of 20. Relax and raise the upper body gradually to a standing position.

Turn and repeat on the other side. Count to 20 for each phase on each side.

Level: Beginners may not be able to fully straighten the leg in the second phase. Extend slowly until a gentle tension is felt.

Comments: Ensure that the rear knee is raised off the floor in the first phase. Keep the spine straight, exhale, and do not bounce. Take care to not stand up too quickly.

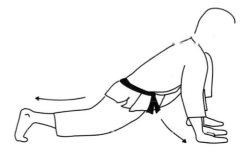

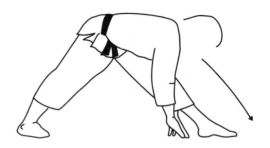

Knee Rotations

Stance: Stand with feet together.

Action: Bend the knees and reach down with heel of hands to stabilize kneecaps. Begin with small slow circles of the knees, spiralling outward into a larger rotation that includes movements of the ankles.

Duration: Ten circles in each direction.

Comments: Observe the shift of body weight from toes to sides of feet and heels. Ensure that both feet are receiving an equal and balanced load.

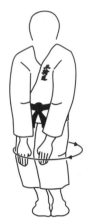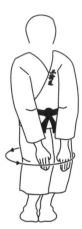

Groin Stretch

Stance: Sit comfortably on the floor with spine straight, legs open, and feet two shoulder widths apart.

Action: Bend knees and grasp one ankle at a time to bring both feet toward groin with the soles together. Let your elbows drop to the inside of the thighs and push slowly down, leaning the body slightly forward until you feel a gentle tension. Hold for a count of ten, then relax the position.

For the next phase, reach forward to grasp feet above the ankles again. With spine straight, pull upward on the ankles and pull your chest forward toward the feet. Exhale and hold for a count of ten at the point of gentle tension.

Level: For more advanced elongation, bring feet closer to the groin.

Comments: Pay careful attention to keeping the spine straight and eyes looking forward.

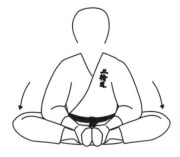

Leg and Lower Back

Stance: Sit with legs apart in front of you.

Action: Bring heel of right foot in toward the groin. Turn upper body to face the extended left leg and, grasping this leg, pull the chest down toward the knee.

Keep the spine straight and neck and head in line with spine. Exhale and hold at the point of gentle tension. Relax and repeat on the other side.

Duration: Count to 20 for each leg.

Level: Variations may include pointing toes or fully flexing them in order to engage different muscle groups in calf or thigh.

Comments: For the basic exercise, feet should be relaxed but with toes pointing up on the extended leg. Do not lower head to knee, but rather feel that you are pulling chest to knee.

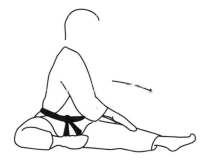

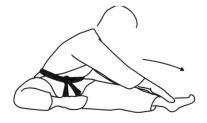

Legs Open and Drop Chest, Side

Stance: Sit on the floor, spine straight, legs open and relaxed, without locking or bending the knees.

Action: Rotate the chest toward left leg and let the chest drop gently to the knee in a down and forward motion. Grasp the leg sufficiently to hold the stance, not to pull. Progressively, reach first for the thigh, then the knee, followed by the shin and finally the ankle. Those who desire an extra stretch should reach beyond the foot and clasp both hands in front of the sole of the foot.

Look toward the foot and elongate the spine. The action will be noticeable on the back of the legs and lower back. The degree of difficulty will increase with opening of the legs. Exhale as you drop the torso, then maintain a comfortable breathing rhythm. Hold the stance for at least four complete breaths. Repeat on the other side.

Comments: Pay careful attention to keeping the spine straight and head up, and do not bounce.

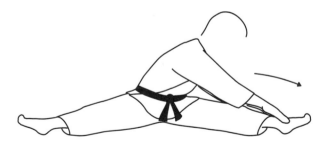

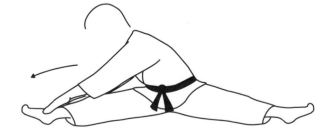

Legs Open and Drop Chest, Center

Stance: Sit on the floor, spine straight, legs wide open and relaxed, without locking or bending the knees.

Action: Slide both hands forward until you feel a gentle stretch in the groin. Hold this position for four breaths. Then flex elbows toward the ground and drop the chest in a forward and down direction to elongate the back. Hold the stance and breathe four cycles more. Once this position is comfortable, slide the hands a bit forward and repeat the action of the breathing and hold cycle.

Look forward, keeping your head in line with your spine. The degree of difficulty will increase with the opening of the legs. Exhale when you lower the torso but do not hold the breath. Establish a comfortable breathing rhythm. Back off the stretch a little bit if breathing is difficult. Hold the stance for at least four complete breaths.

Comments: Pay careful attention to keeping the spine straight. When holding the extended positions and increasing the degree of difficulty, support the weight of your upper body on the hands, otherwise the back muscles will act in tension and it will be counterproductive to their elongation. If you can lower the chest to the ground without forcing it, the stance and the breathing becomes very relaxed and refreshing.

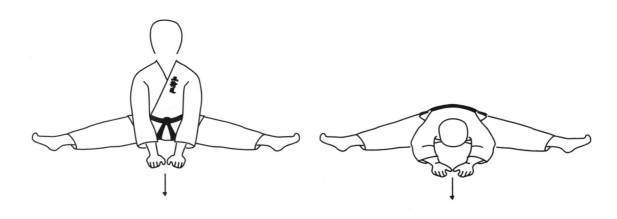

Hip and Lower Back

Stance: Lie on the back, legs extended, and hands at side.

Action: Slowly raise left knee to chest and grasp hands around shin. Pull leg in toward chest and hold, exhaling slowly for a count of ten. Keep spine straight and opposite hip and thigh flat on the floor for maximum benefit.

For phase two, cross the bent knee to the opposite (right) side, with the thigh at a 90° angle to the length of the body, and pull the knee gently down *toward* the floor with the right hand. Do not try to reach the floor with the knee if this alters spine alignment. Keep both shoulders on the floor and allow the back to turn gently. Exhale and hold for a count of ten. Return knee to chest and hold again for a count of ten. Relax and extend leg. Repeat on other side. When changing legs, fully extend the leg just bent before bending the new one. Avoid having both legs in the air at the same time as this can overload the lower spine. All movements should be done slowly.

Comments: Pay close attention to your spine and hip alignment. The point of the first part of this exercise is not to raise the knee as high or close as you can. If the upper thigh lifts from the floor and the spine bends, the target muscle is not being stretched. Relax the rest of your body and breathe comfortably.

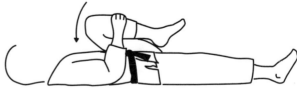

Dog Stretch

Stance: Kneel, with hands shoulder width apart on floor in front of you.

Action: Shift weight to hands, straighten legs and raise hips to form an inverted V, with head down and spine straight. With heels on the floor, feel the gentle tension in the back of both calves. Exhale, continuing breathing, and count to ten.

Alternately bend one knee in a relaxed manner to feel the pull on the opposite calf. Count to ten on each side. When finished, return to kneeling position then slowly curl up your spine, raising head and eyes last.

Comments: Maintain relaxed position of the head in line. Don't hyperextend the straight knee.

Exercise caution when standing up from the kneeling position. Move slowly to avoid a dizzy reaction to blood rushing from the head.

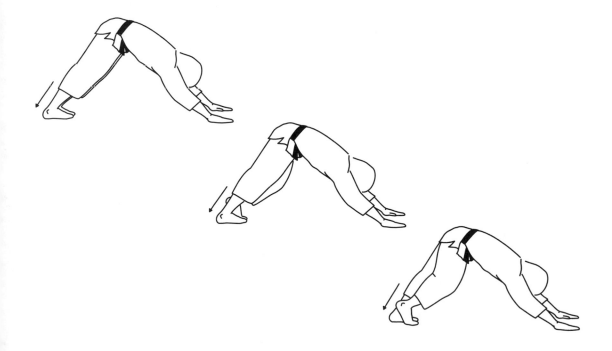

Secrets of the Martial Arts

- A martial artist will gain an understanding of the goal of flexibility early in his practice; for the martial artist, flexibility unites strength with the ability to yield, both mentally and physically.

- Satisfaction rather than gratification must be the goal of the martial arts student, who will take many small steps before being able to map progress with landmarks.

- After a period of inactivity or injury, caution must be exercised to slowly retrain or refresh the body and its integration with the mind.

- The advanced student will look forward to learning something new, and not be overly concerned with the mistakes that will be made as part of that learning process.

- A martial art is a discipline that stresses excellence. This pursuit, however, is one that is acquired through dedication and is not necessarily one that comes naturally.

- The *dojo* is not a special place by itself, but becomes special because of the attitude and training of the people in it.

- A training session always begins with good warm-up, exercises that gently loosen the muscles and joints and gradually proceed to larger movements that raise the body temperature.

- Flexibility in martial arts begins in the mind, is led by the will, and nurtured by the breathing. It has to be understood as an improved arrangement of the body segments that allows for fluid mobility without strain.

- It is more important to achieve a functional state of balanced readiness than the occasional extreme state of high performance.

- One should stretch only when the muscles are fully warm and to an extent appropriate for the level of activity performed that day.

- The secret to maximizing the strength and power to deliver blows, and the speed to avoid blows, lies in the turning movement of the hips.

- Relying on strength alone to resist an assault can lead to defeat when you are faced with someone bigger and stronger, or when injured, sick or aged, or simply when your opponent knows how to use your own force against you.

Chapter 5

Vital Points, to Heal and Protect

EVERYTHING flows from *ki*. This vital energy circulates in the body and throughout our living environment. It may, in fact, be what makes the universe expand. It may also be what holds it all together. Known as *chi* to the Chinese, the concept of *ki* (as it is called in both Japanese and Korean) has both physical and spiritual dimensions. Although much studied, *ki* remains somewhat mysterious and difficult to define precisely in Western terms, even though it is the central principle in Eastern healing arts that have been practiced for millenia.

Although aspects of what we understand as *ki* are variously described in the West as life-force, living energy, atomic attraction, and even the holy spirit, they are typically downplayed because they are not easily quantified, isolated, and tested. We speak of individuals having intestinal fortitude, survival instinct, or internal energy, but we don't know where it comes from, what it is, or how to control it. We glory in the wonders of nature and yet position our species as separate from trees, flowers, and even other members of the animal world. We Westerners prefer to treat all knowledge as specialized and compartmentalized. How the human body works on a molecular level and how planets orbit the sun we consider two completely unrelated areas of inquiry. Yet scientists who have probed deeply in these seemingly opposite directions have discovered bewildering similarities, and phenomena that defy current explanation and codification. Although the scientific method does not generally allow for the existence of anything outside of that which can be tested, with results independently duplicated, many great discoveries have occurred by accident, or by the adventurous mind that was not afraid to ask "what if?"

In the long history of Eastern culture, adherence to this scientific method has not presented the same problems in the search for knowledge and understanding. By recognizing and building from concepts of integration and synergy, these societies have generated quite a different approach to how the human organism and spirit interact. Eastern religions, educational methods, healing arts, and even political systems have, traditionally at least, been more holistic, circular, and long lasting than many of the dogmas and technologies of the West. While we

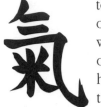

Ki: *energy, or spirit*

tend to not accept or believe something until it has been explained or proven "scientifically," Eastern practice has been to follow what works, and study it on that level. Because of these different ways of thinking, it is only recently that Western medicine and science have paid respect to the Eastern healing practices. Relatively little scientific study has been done of acupuncture, for example, yet the medical profession moved quickly in many state legislatures to limit those who could practice it, claiming it constituted a risk to the public. Generally, there has been little financial support for rigorous testing of acupuncture and other *ki* healing therapies, including herbal remedies, although some exploratory work has been done. One has to question the motivation of a medical establishment that invests billions of dollars in pharmaceutical interests, and which might significantly be affected by drugless therapies for the treatment of pain, chronic illness, and depression. Never mind the consequences if early studies bear out the indication that acupuncture can effectively aid in quitting smoking. We can only hope that as communication improves, awareness expands and eyes are opened, that the knowledge gathered in these now separate systems can be shared, and lead to the opening of many new windows on the human condition. It will be unfortunate if the insecurities of the establishment were allowed to slow the progress of learning and discovery.

Despite years of study, testing, and dissection of animals and the human body, scientists have not been able to tell us what life precisely is. We know when life exists and when it does not exist anymore, and we have an elaborate definition of what constitutes a life form. Nevertheless, Western science or medicine has not been able to give us a model with anywhere near the elegance of that of *ki* or *chi*.

Ki is generated internally in living things but also flows through them and their environment. This life energy is all important to an Eastern understanding of health and healing. Any disruption in the flow or balance of *ki* is thought to lead to sickness, and the aim of most treatment systems is to restore this flow and strengthen the mechanisms by which it is balanced or amplified. This relationship of *ki* as a healing energy is fundamental to Eastern medicine, which recognizes

Locations of Ki Centers (chakras)

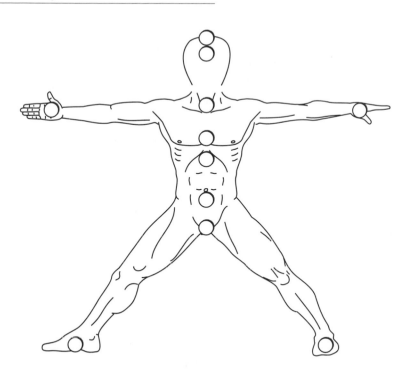

that ultimately the body-mind heals itself. Even Western medicine reluctantly admits that despite its technology, drugs, and surgical refinements, patients must still do their own healing.

Ki energy and its power are intimately connected with breathing. As we have discussed, breathing fuels the furnace of internal energy and regulates its circulation. For the Chinese this process has developed into a field of of study and practice known as *chi kung*, where techniques of breathing and developing the focus of *chi* are used for healing, strengthening, and transmission of energy. The modern movement exercises of *tai chi chuan* are manifestations of this study, and are practiced to maintain and improve health. Although not as readily recognized by the Western public as a martial art, *tai chi chuan* uses the knowledge of energy, focus, and breathing for self-protection and redirection of the energy of an attack.

Acupuncture and herbal medicine also manipulate and restore the proper functioning of the *chi. Shiatsu, sotai, reiki,* and *kiatsu* are the most well known of the healing arts from the Japanese line that are based on the *ki* concept.

Martial artists are also learning how to develop and channel their *ki* and how to adapt to the *ki* of others. Defensively, one can think of deflecting the energy of an opponent's attack, disrupting its flow, or blocking or overpowering another's *ki* with one's own. Primarily, the practitioner is concerned with his own *ki* and is taught to be balanced and centered within that energy.

The important *ki* center for the martial artist is the *tanden*, often referred to as the *hara*. This center is located approximately three finger widths below the navel, and the middle interior, of the body. Students focus their mind on breathing from this spot when practicing *zazen* and are exhorted continually to let their energy flow directly from this zone as they learn movement technique.

To the Japanese, the *hara* is more than the physiological connection that we interpret from the *ki* centers of the healing arts. There are psychological and spiritual components that relate to the character of the martial artist and have to do with strength, will, and intention. *Hara*, which is sometimes loosely translated as "belly," can be used to describe "attitude," which in the West we might refer to as "intestinal fortitude" or "guts." One is said to have *hara* when conducting oneself in a brave, dignified manner. There is a strong sense of calm, hidden power associated with the term in Japanese culture, and it is central to views of morality, leadership, and duty.

There is a physical aspect that relates to these images as well, that of being at equilibrium or in balance, with a low center of gravity. As we have discussed previously, Western body images locate the center of gravity much higher in the body, and similarly, the important emotional motivation is said to be the heart. Overdevelopment of the upper body through weightlifting is still a common error in sports programs and home exercise regimes. Athletes who succeed in sports requiring balance and agility, however, are tending toward a lowering of their mass, and building strength in the legs and abdomen with a relaxed upper body is their training goal. This is one of the areas where professional sports have looked to the martial arts for guidance. Skiers, figure skaters, and hockey players, for example, are literally turning the tables on previously conceived notions of body type and development to achieve excellence in their sports. Dancers are more athletic, and gymnasts and divers look different at elite levels than they did a decade ago. Nevertheless, many athletes, especially women, still suffer from derogatory descriptions like "thunder thighs" and "peasant's calf" when described by media and spectators. It may be some time before our standards of beauty are modified to reflect health and fitness values, rather than the anorexic look of runway models.

Moving and breathing from the *hara* is fundamental to good technique that has power, focus, and control. Utilizing this *ki* center of energy is a practice that is cultivated in both the martial and healing arts. The martial artist learns to access and release his reserves of energy and to concentrate that strength in a specific place, at a specific moment.

Three Examples of Meridians

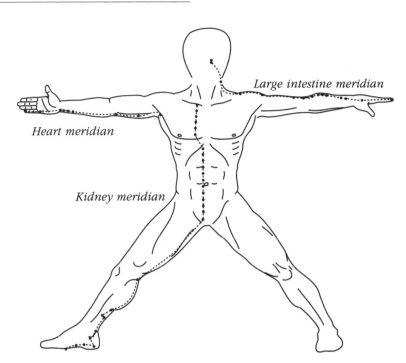

Large intestine meridian

Heart meridian

Kidney meridian

Acupuncturists and others working with *ki* also learn to direct this energy, their own and that of their patients, both for restoring the flow of healthy energy and eliminating toxins from the body. The martial arts share this knowledge and understanding of *ki*, and in small villages in Asia the healers were traditionally martial artists. This function, along with the transformation of energy from the control of breathing, and the utilization of *ki* energy for power, is most applicable to the martial artist of today.

The exchange of *ki* with our surroundings takes place through the air we breathe and the food we eat, as well as the primal configuration of *ki* that we obtained from our parents. *Ki* circulates in the body in channels, usually referred to as meridians. These do not correspond with nerve fibers or blood vessels, but follow their own pathways, often near the surface of the skin. There are numerous locations along these meridians, like stations on a train line, where the flow of *ki* can be accessed; these points can be manipulated with the pressure of the fingers, or finely tuned by the application of fine acupuncture needles, heat, moxibustion, and more recently, laser beams.

The main meridians are organized in *yin* and *yang* pairs corresponding to organ systems of the body. The kidney or heart channels, for example, do not just include the specific organ itself, but also the processes controlled or affected by that organ. There are additional channels to these, two of which, plus the twelve organ channels, make up the fourteen meridians and 361 acupuncture points of classical study. There are more systems, points, and groupings than these for the purpose of categorization, working relationships, and methods of learning acupuncture theory. Axis points, connecting channels, and their interrelations serve to complicate the picture for beginners and outsiders.

There is also a relationship between *ki* centers and the *chakras* of the body that we associate with systems of yoga. These focal points for energy and balancing are mapped by ancient knowledge as well, and have roots in India even earlier than that of the studies of *chi* in China. Breathing, relaxation, and internal strength of spirit are practiced focusing on the *chakras*. Many spiritual and religious traditions have evolved from this knowledge and are well represented in historical texts and artistic traditions.

It is important for us to remember that in Eastern philosophy and health practices, mind and body do not suffer from being thought of as completely distinct and different. Mind, body, and spirit are inextricably wound together when we consider the energy of *ki*. Moreover, the connection of the individual to the circular forces and elements at work in nature is part of this picture. These relationships are important to the study of martial arts and are revealed systematically as one's training proceeds. By practicing the physical, and developing the connections between the conscious and unconscious, the mental and spiritual realities of this energy can begin to be understood. As the skills develop and experience grows, the ability to access and utilize these energies improves. At more advanced levels, the attention turns to *ki* as the primary concern of the practice, and physical technique becomes more of the consequence of the application of *ki*. The reaction becomes the action in this case.

Martial artists understand practically and intuitively that there is more going on in their training than merely the physical. Knowing that the human body is so fragile that it can be easily be damaged should dispel any illusions of invincibility. When practicing, emphasis is on mutual respect and care for the training partner, and this consideration for others is extended outside the walls of the *dojo*.

This ancient knowledge of *ki* is also of interest to martial artists for its own sake, with respect to personal healing, stress relief, and pain management, but also because of the relationship to vital points on the body that can be used for self-defense. There are many points which, if manipulated a certain way, can cause pleasant sensations and healing energies, but if struck or squeezed can cause pain, paralysis, or in some cases, serious injury and death. Throughout the centuries of

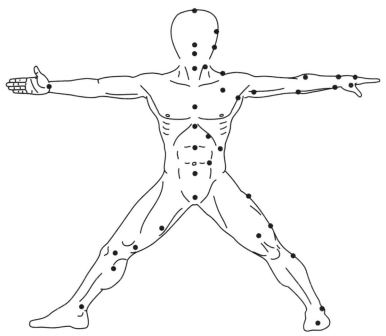

*Vital points for the application of techniques in the martial arts
can be seen to relate to meridians and chakras.*

studying these vital points, there have been various mappings, using drawings or statues, to illustrate the locations of meridians and points. Three-dimensional bronze sculptures were known to have been made as early as 1026 A.D. in China for the purpose of teaching acupuncture and moxibustion students.

In different geographical areas and textual renderings, the same points and their connecting meridians sometimes have different names, presumably to control dissemination of this knowledge to ensure that it was used for appropriate purposes. Certainly acupuncturists are cautioned against the use of certain points, or specific points at certain times, because of the danger of causing injury. In addition, other points were kept as secrets within the ranks of physicians and scholars of the healing and martial arts. It is thought that this knowledge of striking vital points, along with their use in grappling, was introduced in Japan by a Chinese martial artist named Chen Gen Pin who arrived in 1638. His students formed separate schools of *jujutsu* incorporating these techniques.

The study of vital points has captured great attention in Western martial arts literature because of the near magical powers this knowledge seems to impart to the practitioners. However, it is the use of *ki* energy, balancing and focus of power, that pertains directly to the training process. From a health and fitness point of view, this where the real "magic" is, the area of the traditional wisdom that is of most value to modern students.

Clearly, there are many targets available on the human body, where it is weak or where vital organs can be impacted. It is interesting that in Eastern martial arts, special attention has historically been paid to locations that can also heal, and often a strike at these points causes temporary reactions such as pain, paralysis, or unconsciousness without resulting in permanent harm. Knowledge of these points is extremely useful considering the "prime directive" of self-defense, that an opportunity to escape or immobilize an attack is always the preferred strategy. The more the martial artist learns about the areas of vulnerability of the human body, the more he becomes aware of having to protect them.

Many of the techniques of the martial arts are not immediately understood by those involved in the sport aspect, where attacks only to certain prescribed zones are allowed, and scoring points given only for blows that land, not those deflected by an effective defense. Stances, and combinations that might deliver the most power in an attack, are often modified to those in which one's own exposure is lessened. Strategically, the martial arts student learns what areas of the body are inherently stronger or less vulnerable, and these targets are sometimes "sacrificed" in defense while others can be moved away from harm. Similarly, openings are created by exposing an obvious vital target, with the intention of luring an opponent's attack and countering the predicted attack with a planned response.

As is true with most living organisms, our important points of vulnerability lie long the center line of the body, the more vulnerable or soft areas being on the front or ventral side. This coincides with the vital targets, accupoints, and *chakras* previously mentioned. It is no coincidence that the guard positions of martial art training seek to defend against attack to the center line while maintaining mobility. Fists, forearms, elbows, knees, and shins are employed as moving screens in front of the center line.

The practice of reflexive technique improves the student's ability to anticipate the direction of attack, and develops the ability to deflect a strike while at the same time rotating the body and limbs in such a way as to insure that another vulnerable zone is not exposed. Beginners work with small targets at first, the surface areas of which are increased, step by small step, to include the whole body at advanced levels of training. There are always plateaus in the cognitive processes where one feels naked and unable to cover all vulnerable zones at once, but eventually the mind, body, and spirit unite to act without thinking, as if by instinct. But every martial artist knows that these "instincts" are carefully honed and tuned by hours and years of practice.

The standard targets of martial art practice are the face, the throat, the solar plexus, the floating ribs, the groin, and the knees. On the back or dorsal side of the body these specific zones for counterattack include the base of the skull, the kidneys, the sacrum, back of the knees, and Achilles tendon. One can see that many of these targets lie along the center line of the body as a whole, or the center of the legs. The sides of the knees are another sensitive area with little protection, as well as the side of the head, particularly the soft skull of the temples on the outside of the eyes. The face has many specific targets, many of which such as the eyes, the philtrum at the base of the nose, and the larynx of the throat, can result in lethal injury if struck with force. In addition to these are all the vital points previously mentioned.

The aim is to throw every bone and muscle of the body wide open so that the chi *may travel unobstructed. Once this is done the chest must be further relaxed and the* chi *made to sink to the navel. After time the* chi *will be felt accumulating for mass integration in the navel, from where it will circulate in the body.*

•

Cheng Man-ch'ing 1902–75

When students realize the great number of targets that must be protected, they pay more attention to their stances, movement, and blocking and worry less about their punches and kicks. When we recognize how easy it is to actually injure or seriously harm someone with all these known targets, we can wonder why one would need a "secret death punch" directed to a "secret death spot." Martial artists learn quickly that their course of study is not about dealing death, but rather the cultivation of their own strength and flexibility in order to defend themselves in the event a fight cannot be avoided. As the martial artist advances, these defenses will utilize more and more of the repertoire of vital points and sensitive areas by use of controlling, neutralizing, and immobilizing techniques that involve the minimum of force.

In stretching exercises or the hyperextension of joints during the manipulation of self-defense techniques, the practitioner must quickly recognize the difference between the "sweet discomfort" of extension of muscles and ligaments, and the pain of damaging stress on these tissues. Students are taught when first working with partners to "tap out" a safety signal before this type of pain presents itself. This safety tap is rigorously respected, and in addition to preventing injury in practice, teaches a sensitivity that helps refine the location, angle, and intensity of the application of technique. The martial artist becomes very adept at quickly finding the weak point of an attack and defending against it using minimum effort. Being effective is a primary goal of martial arts training, whether this involves a pressure point, a joint lock, a deflecting blow, or a preemptive strike. We can see here again the importance of the strict traditions of the *dojo*. Without the trust and control of technique that comes from proper attitude, good instruction, and careful supervision, as well as friendly respect for the training partner, such subtle skills cannot be learned, because they cannot be practiced.

By combining this type of knowledge with an understanding of how to stay relaxed when falling, rolling on hard surfaces, twisting to distribute the impact of a blow over a larger surface area, and exhaling when absorbing impact, a martial artist possesses tools that can prevent or minimize injury in an accident situation. Many practitioners have avoided or survived automotive, skiing, and biking accidents, for example, by reacting with the skills of their training.

There are also equally dramatic stories of martial artists using their breathing, focus, visualization, and relaxation techniques to recover from serious illness, or injuries requiring long rehabilitation periods. Western medical professionals have often been surprised by the recoveries of martial artist patients in their care, and have attributed their speed to their conditioning and mental determination. Eastern physicians would, of course, understand this more readily, and often are more able to work successfully with martial artists because of their knowledge of *ki* energy, their ability to concentrate, and their patience.

Martial artists have been interested in the use of herbal remedies, massage, and *ki* therapies as long as they have been training. Some traditional training styles and more advanced levels of practice involve such intensive training that the massage of sore muscles, the realignment of joints, neck and spine, and soothing treatments for bruises and blisters is, of course, most welcome. Older schools incorporated the teaching of techniques to set broken bones, methods of resuscitation,

Koichi Tohei Principles of Ki Exercise

- Movements center on and begin from the One Point in the lower abdomen.
- *Ki* is fully extended in each movement.
- Move freely and easily.
- Do not feel any tension in the muscles.
- Show and feel a clear sense of rhythm in your movements.

from *Ki: A Road that Anyone Can Walk*
by William Reed

and even reanimation for those more seriously injured. This knowledge came from experience on the battlefield, and led later to the tradition of martial artists, possessing such useful knowledge of the human body, being asked to step in when more specialized medical help was unavailable.

Today's martial artists and athletes in general are more knowledgeable about the immediate treatment of injuries, and how to relate their physical training to their rehabilitation from them. Most sports medicine specialists and trauma physicians in general acknowledge that the sooner an injury is attended to, even by the simple application of ice, compression, and elevation, the greater the chance of reducing damage and complications, accelerating healing, and restoring mobility.

As the training of a martial artist progresses, he learns to distinguish between the signals of different types of pain and discomfort. For example, between the burning sensation of oxygen debt or lactic acid build-up in muscle and the pain of muscle tears, shin splits, or tendonitis from the overuse of a joint. While the latter conditions signal impending injury and indicate that a slowing or cessation of activity is necessary, the former will be recognized as temporary, and ameliorated by careful practice, a good cool-down, and sometimes just a hot bath or self-massage after the practice session.

Most martial artists acknowledge that they experience fewer injuries, get sick less often, and recover more quickly as they become more advanced in their training. Children, especially, find that their health is improved, they are less susceptible to infections, and conditions such as asthma, (which in the past were contraindicated for vigorous activities), are actually much improved and in some cases cured, by participation in the martial arts.

Advanced martial artists tend to be drawn to healing practices that reflect the principles upon which their bodies and minds have been aligned, and to which they have grown to feel more spiritually complementary. As their awareness of the function of their own bodies improves and becomes more sensitive, they demand that their health professionals respect their opinions and work hand in hand to preserve their health. Martial artists can and should utilize their inherent strength and flexibility when dealing with sicknesses or injuries. As their training becomes more centered on the understanding and use of *ki*, so will the rest of their daily lives.

One Wrist Rotation, Outside to Inside

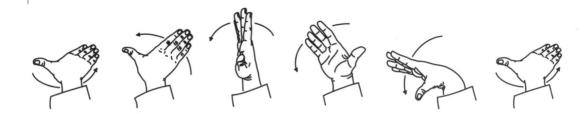

Action: Rotation of the wrist facilitates strength and flexibility of the joint and improves circulation in the hand and arm. It is also a fundamental self-defense response reflex.

As a health exercise, this rotation can be practiced at any time in any position. It should be done slowly, seeking each time a line of movement free of tension or interruption. Feel as if you are "breathing through the fingers," and exhale slowly with slight pressure as you complete each circle. Repeat five times.

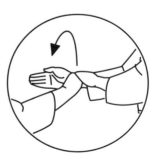

Comments: In the application of the wrist rotation as a self-defense technique, pressure is applied against an opponent's wrist that causes him to let go, due to pain or disruption of the grappling strength. One can see in the examples on the right that these techniques are directed at pressure points that can cause weakness when applied with force, but when practiced with a partner can stimulate *ki* centers and activate meridians that promote health.

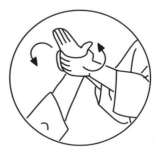

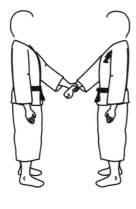
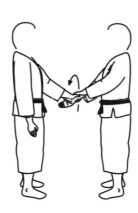
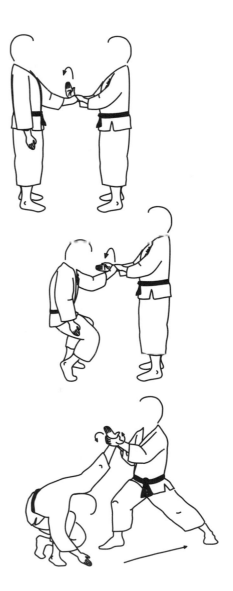

This example presents a defense against someone grabbing the wrist on the same side. The defender clasps the attacker's hand to immobilize it against his own. He then rotates his hand in a small outside-to-inside circle. The objective is to bring the outside edge of the heel of his hand against the same place on the opponent's (where the hand meets the wrist). Acting with a gentle pressure on the opponent's wrist joint, ligaments, and tendons, the rest of his body can be put out of balance, impeding any possible counterattack. As a defense this motion is very short and direct. It can be finished by controlling the wrist joint completely by bringing the other hand to the repositioning of the attack. Exhale when applying pressure and keep the elbows close to the side of the body.

One Wrist Rotation, Inside to Outside

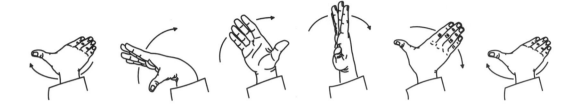

Action: The movement of the hand and wrist in this exercise is similar to the previous one but in the opposite direction. Done slowly and without tension, this rotation exercise can increase mobility in the wrist. Exhale through to completion of the circle. Repeat five times.

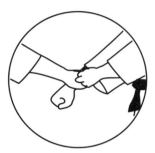

Comments: In these close-ups of the full self-defense technique on the opposite page we can see how knowledge of vital points and their connections facilitates the application of technique, in addition to the simple locking of the joints against their natural range of movement. The gentle practice of these techniques can have beneficial effects on the students, stimulating *ki* points and nerve centers as well as massaging and stretching joints, muscles, and meridians.

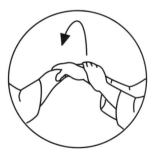

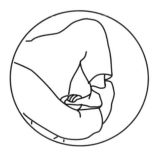

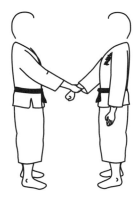 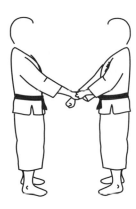 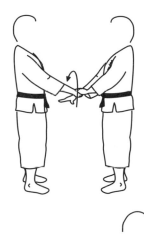

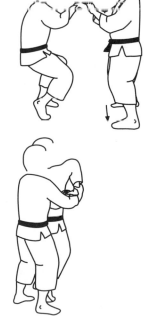

This self-defense technique is a response to a grab of the wrist on the opposite side, crossing the body. The defender immediately responds with a knuckle strike to the middle of the back of the hand of the attacker. This strike will distract the attacker and, if accurately applied, will loosen the grip, even to the point of temporarily paralyzing the attacker's hand. The striking hand then moves to grasp and immobilize the opponent's hand against his own wrist. The defender continues with an inside-to-outside rotation, grasping the inside of the opponents wrist with his fingers. Slight pressure from closing of the hand will unbalance the opponent. By moving behind the opponent and shifting the position of the hands to bend the fingers up and behind, the opponent can be persuaded to "come along" and discontinue his attack.

Secrets of the Martial Arts

- *Ki* is generated internally in living things but also flows through them and their environment. This life energy is all important to Eastern understanding of health and healing.

- Martial artists are also learning how to develop and channel their *ki* and how to adapt to the *ki* of others.

- Primarily, the practitioner is concerned with his own *ki* and is taught to be balanced and centered within using that energy.

- Moving and breathing from the *hara* is fundamental to the development of good technique that has power, focus, and control. Utilizing this *ki* center of energy is a practice that is cultivated in both the martial and healing arts.

- Mind, body, and spirit are inextricably wound together when we consider the energy of *ki*. Moreover, the connection of the individual to the circular forces and elements at work in nature is part of this picture.

- This ancient knowledge is of interest to martial artists for its own sake with respect to personal healing, stress relief, and pain management, but also because of the relationship to vital points of the body that can be used for self-defense.

- The more the martial artist learns about all the areas of vulnerability of the human body, the more he is aware of having to protect them.

- As is true with most living organisms, our important points of vulnerability lie along the center line of the body, the more vulnerable or soft areas being on the front, or ventral, side.

- The martial artist becomes very adept at quickly finding the weak point of an attack and defending against it, using minimum effort.

- Most martial artists acknowledge that they experience fewer injuries, get sick less often, and recover more quickly as they become more advanced in their training.

- Advanced martial artists tend to be drawn to healing practices that reflect the principles upon which their bodies and minds have been aligned, and which have grown to feel spiritually complementary.

Chapter 6

Harmony of Energy, Kiai

WHEN the tiger roars, the dog barks, or the cat meows, it is only their *kiai* that awakens you. By summoning the internal energy of *ki*, focusing it with our mind and releasing it with our spirit, we also can create *kiai*. The word literally means a "union of energy," but we are more familiar with its external, vocal expression. The *kiai*, or spirit yell, is the loud percussive shout that is given off by martial artists when they train.

Although every *kiai* is unique, it is formed by the forceful expulsion of air from deep within the lungs. It is propelled by the diaphragm muscle and the contraction of the abdomen, and shaped by the glottis and voice box of the larnyx. Usually loud and startling, the *kiai* is tempered by the situation and the "feel" of the moment. Depending on the technique being applied, the *kiai* shout may be short or long, pitched high or low, joyful or fierce. The varied timbres of this voice have been described as having seasons—spring, fall, winter, summer—and are modified according to changes in internal energy.

The real *kiai*, of course, is the union of energy itself; the shout is only its manifestation. This is sometimes forgotten by martial artists, especially when using a *kiai* in a *kata* to attract attention and present a particular image for the performance in tournament. Like the "canned" *kiai* from the soundtracks of martial arts movies, these shouts sound fake at best, and are usually exaggerated to the point of providing much fodder for those who would make fun of "kung fu fighters." Imitation of movie heroes or wild animals, or yelling for the sake of yelling does not constitute a *kiai*. A real *kiai* must be honest, uninhibited, and a pure expression of spirit; only then is it useful to the martial artist.

As we discussed in the last chapter, it is by the cultivation and application of energy that a martial artist becomes truly powerful. By improving the balance of *ki* we become healthier, and as a source of energy when training, *ki* allows our body fabric to become strong, limber, and tuned to the demands placed on it by our mental processes. However, it is truly when our spirit is kindled, and integrated with the physical and intellectual elements of the training, that *ki* begins to work for us.

Kiai is present always in the martial artist. It should not be identified only with states of excitement or exertion, for it can be called upon at rest to calm the mind and body, and when weak or injured, to rejuvenate and recuperate. The student begins to learn *kiai* when composing himself before bowing at the *dojo* door, and again when exhaling the first breath in *zazen*. By bringing himself in union with the moment and then with the internal, *ki* has been brought "on-line." We have mentioned how extraordinary situations have forced individuals to summon great energy for survival or defense, or the creation of works of art. The martial artist seeks to access and utilize this reservoir of power in his training, and be able to direct it in meaningful ways.

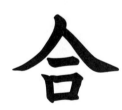

Kiai: *union of energy*

The audible expression of *kiai* is a tool that can serve many purposes. It is usually first practiced as an exercise to ensure that the student is engaging his diaphragm and expanding his lungs for abdominal breathing. By using the voice and the gentle contraction of the throat to close off the windpipe, a small back pressure can be created. The student tries to coordinate the release of this air with the contraction of the abdomen in a forced expulsion. For a beginner, shouting the word *kiai* can assist in this action, because of the shapes that the oral cavity must form to say it; the air builds up behind the "k" and is released with the "yai." As the student progresses, the *kiai* will become more natural and individual, and won't necessarily be formed as any particular word, because the throat must be relaxed to allow the energy to come from within. A *kiai* that is too high in the throat is ineffective, and results in soreness and fatigue of the voice. Senior students and teachers are also taught to use this relaxed voice form of *kiai* when counting and giving commands to the group, in order to convey energy and establish timing without fatiguing the voice.

When the student learns to coordinate the sound with the exhalation of air, he begins to use *kiai* when strength or effort is required, as in lifting or striking. Most people are familiar with a martial artist using a *kiai* when punching, kicking, or breaking a board. The *kiai* is a common tool used to assist in the power and focus of these techniques. In this case he is directing his *ki* toward a point in space. He will focus this energy using *kiai*, (verbally as well) to create *kime*, which is the maximum expression of energy in the minimum time.

Let us look at the act of breaking a one-inch pine board as both a practical demonstration and also as a metaphor for the concept of *kime*. A physicist will explain that the board is composed of numerous fibers of cellulose, layered and bound together with a certain tensile strength and rigidity depending on its species and age of the wood. These fibers are composed of molecules of carbon, hydrogen, and oxygen, bound together by the electrical energy of their chemical components. At the level of the hard board and the soft hand rising to meet it, science will explain that if sufficient energy is applied in a small area, it can break these bonds.

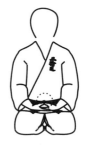

It is really not that difficult to break a board or brick this way, if the blow is accurate, the speed high, and the kinetic energy directed *through* the hard surface. In the case of boards and blocks piled one on top of another it is the same force breaking the surface that is transferred and transmitted through the layers underneath. The energy and compression of the impact are directed into the board, not back into the flesh and bone of the hand. As it turns out, bone as a physical substance is quite dense, strong, and somewhat forgiving, if the force is applied correctly. What primarily breaks a board though, is accuracy and speed.

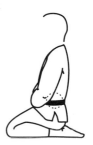

However, there is much more to these exercises for a martial artist. Board-breaking is not simply a trick to please crowds, but useful in training *kime*, because in addition to the physical and mental, the spiritual dimension begins to enter the picture. The student must *believe* that the board will break and his hand pass through unharmed. He must be able to visualize this experience without pain or stoppage, or the board will not break and it will hurt, a lot. By understanding the physical principles, translating them through the body, calling upon the coordination of this energy to create a technique that flows, with a focal point beyond the board, the board will part like tall grass in the wind. There is no magic here, but force of will and intention are just as much part of the concept of *kime* as surface tension and the vectors of applied force.

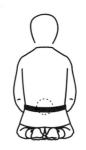

The location of the hara.

The *kiai* is useful for many other aspects of martial art training and self-defense. As we have said, the most fundamental skill is control of the breath. When confronted with a frightening situation, the breathing mechanism can become paralyzed. The typical victim in the horror movie who immediately brings his knuckles to his mouth and screams, is actually in better shape than most, because with the prolonged exhalation of the scream, breathing is restored, oxygen circulates, and

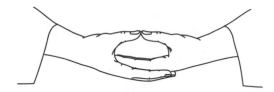

Hand position in seiza, *"Neither valley nor mountain."*

fainting is avoided. The martial art student is taught the *kiai* as the first response to a strike, hold, or grab. Most people think that the conditioning of this reflex is for the purpose of startling and distracting the attacker, and while it does serve this purpose, it is more important to help maintain breathing, strength levels, and to keep his wits together. Studies have shown that grip strength and mental faculties decrease rapidly when the breath is held. It is vital for the martial artist to be able to keep moving, and have access to his energy and skills in an emergency situation. An automatic *kiai* helps him do this.

Similarly, the *kiai* can be used in less threatening circumstances: to shake off nervousness, reduce blood pressure, or adjust attitude quickly when faced with feelings of panic or anxiety. A good bark can usually make an attacking animal (human or canine) back off with their tail between their legs. A well developed *kiai* can alert someone across a street of imminent danger, break a crystal goblet, or start an avalanche, but primarily the martial artist uses it in his regular training sessions to summon and sustain his energy. A *kiai* will signal the start or end of a technique or a series of repetitions. It is used to communicate a change in direction in *kihon* (basic drills), or readiness to answer an attack in *ippon kumite* (one-step, pre-arranged sparring). When one is fatigued or exhausted, a few good *kiai* can awaken and revitalize oneself or a training partner. Particularly in long sessions where the student feels the limits of endurance have been reached, second, third, and even fourth winds can be "kick started" by a deep *kiai*. Group training with simultaneous *kiai* can make the room shake and muscles quiver.

Although there is anecdotal evidence of martial artists using *kiai* to break glass, knock over opponents, and even kill from a distance, the source and effect of *kiai*, both intrinsic and expressed, is a positive one. There are accounts of breathing and pulse being restored when a martial arts healer has used a *kiai*. Like a good belly laugh or three cheers for a jolly good fellow, the *kiai* is a joyful noise unto the universe. In its pure form it connects the individual with his soul and that lonely soul with something greater.

This concept of *kiai*, associated with the instantaneous idea of *kime*, relates to explosive power. But it is equally important to remember that *kiai* should also be accessed as a creative energy, in relaxed flowing movement, subtle finesses, and strong sustained efforts. *Kiai* is predominantly related to the spirit of the practitioner, but has to be equally connected to the physical and mental, to become the union of energy that powers martial art practice. In three-step sparring, or combinations that employ three successive steps, the student is taught to organize himself in a progression that leads to the *kiai*. The first step represents the body, the second the mind, with its contradictions and limitations, and the third, the spirit, without limitation and fully expressed, which is *kiai*.

Kiai holds the emotional content favored by the martial artist. Transforming or redirecting anger, fear, and frustration into the joy of *kiai* allows the student to penetrate beyond the superficial and work toward a mastery of the self that is individual and enlightened. This *kiai*, when centered physically and psychologically in the *hara*, allows the martial artist to stride quietly through his world with great energy. This feeling is very physical. When training *kihon*, running in the woods, or spinning through a *kata*, the practitioner floats in his body, like sitting on a horse that is sensitive to every thought and intention of its rider. This perception of the *hara* flows from the first lessons about breathing, bowing, and standing. The mental image of a samurai posing comfortably atop the wide breadth of his warrior horse is often evoked to convey the feeling of relaxed power. Later in the training, as the ability to rotate the hips and to direct technique from the *hara* improves, the student becomes more aware of the flow of strength and well-being emanating from this area.

The power of *kiai* will sustain the martial artist through periods of fatigue and weakness, as well as grief, frustration, or despair. These physical and psychological states are co-dependent and intertwined with corresponding opposite states such as energetic joy and irrepressible zeal. As a pendulum swings between these extremes it passes through a center point where eventually, if no other force acted upon it, it would come to rest, in the same way a set of scales will tilt back and forth about a central fulcrum. As we have seen, a balanced *ki* or centered *hara* has more to do with balance in motion than at rest. The body sitting in *zazen* has a very difficult time staying still. The whisper of a breeze, even a passing thought, will shift the mental and physical balance.

A better symbolic image for the *kiai* of the martial artist is riding a bicycle, where balance is acquired by the motion of the wheels and

Spirit (ki) . . . *All action is motivated by this creating force.*

A creating consciousness, being internal, and physical action, being external, can best be put to the optimum if they are coordinated into perfect harmony of thought and motion. This spirit, utilizing the maximum of all mental and physical cells and organs is what the masters speak of when they discuss communion of mind and body.

•

Choi Hong Hi
1918—

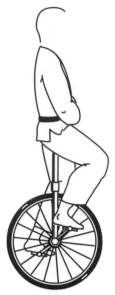

Balance in motion.

the forward propulsion of the body and bicycle. At higher speeds, the effort required to sustain motion, to change direction, or to recover balance, is minimal and subtle. This metaphor is also useful in visualizing and understanding the physical and the mental aspects of the application of *kiai*. We must not lose the image of the calm hub at the center of the spinning wheel, whether we are visualizing circularity of breathing while still sitting in *seiza*, or executing a jumping, spinning kick. At the same time, we want to have a sense of forward motion while exhilarating in the moment. The verbal *kiai* that we build toward in the culmination of a technique is the outward expression, the expansion and release of the internal circularity that fuels our efforts.

The Eastern view of life is a circular passage from birth to death to being born again. This view respects the rhythms of nature and is both physical and spiritual in its science and philosophies. The techniques of martial art use the principles of circulation of energy as well as physical effects, such as centrifugal and centripetal forces. The student is taught to breathe and expand his lungs and mind from a center in *seiza*. He learns to move forward, backward, to each side, and diagonally with equal ease. By doing so he develops a sense of his sphere of influence, and begins to feel like he has "eyes in the back of his head." The usefulness of such awareness in self-defense is obvious, but like most principles in the martial arts, upon further examination, the practical gives way to the philosophical.

In martial arts we refer to this zone, this "bubble," as *ma-ai*. This area is not strictly defined by a fixed distance from the *hara*, but rather is an ever-changing equation of distance and time, based on our perception of our ability to move and act within it. Personal space, or the distance we keep from another, is a concept that varies depending on the individual moods, and by some accounts our culture. We are more willing to allow people we know inside our personal space than strangers. Animals and humans usually keep a cautionary distance between themselves and what is unknown; we are more likely to cross the street to avoid a stranger when it is dark and deserted than we would at midday on a crowded sidewalk.

The *ma-ai* of the martial artist is a matter of instinct, determined by the vibrations we receive from others. If someone is in that space that makes us feel at risk, we act with heightened awareness and readiness. When working with partners in martial arts practice, this sphere of influence interacts with that of others. We learn to sense the *ma-ai* of others (joining, confluence, harmony, emptiness), first throughout the physical extensions of techniques and eventually by judging and feeling the *ki* energy of each other. This sensitivity reaches deeper than the ability to read the external. Understanding the intention of an opponent, whether friend or foe, goes beyond the merely physical.

Strategically, the martial artist does not want to "telegraph" his intentions about his next move. The Zen attitudes of being "fully in the moment" and "thinking by not thinking" may have appealed to the samurai by helping him to act in the present moment without giving away the next. By the same token, in anticipating the moves of another, one has to exercise caution not to be led by an opening move or feint that draws a reaction before the real attack is launched. By reacting to what *is* rather than what you think will be, your response will be more accurate. But you have to be quick.

Intention, like *kime*, and *ma-ai* and *kiai*, can be summed up in an instant, the instant between life and death. All living things are faced with this threshold eventually, but most of us prefer not to contemplate it. To the samurai who was always prepared to greet death, the moment of living was to be experienced fully without regret. With training, death could be faced untainted by fear, reserve, or apprehension. It was believed that coming to the edge of this transformation from life, brought great power and change to an individual. The death poems of those who were facing battle, or preparing for the ritual suicide known as *seppuku*, were given great importance, and revered for the insights of their authors.

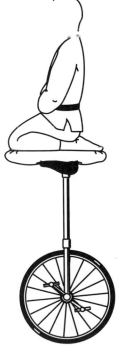

Those who faced death and somehow survived were transformed by their reprieves, as if reborn. This took on traditional meaning in the training of the samurai, and although the practical reality of sudden death became less common as the martial arts developed, the philosophical relationship continued. The student was taught to be fully committed to the training in general, and to each and every technique in particular. The opportunity to be reborn in the execution of a technique, or the deflection of an incoming attack, has a powerful effect on the attitude and spirit of the practitioner. It is important that any single repetition of a technique not be burdened by the success or failure of the one that went before, nor be allowed to bleed into the one coming after. When the excess baggage of frustration, insufficiency, or regret can be put aside, the attention to the training becomes pure and fresh. While this can be extraordinarily difficult, it is critical for

Motionless in balance.

the improvement of the student, and his reconciliation with the process of learning martial art as a voyage rather than a destination.

Another aspect of the re-creation of the life and death struggle that strongly colors the study of the martial arts, is the deep psychological effect of facing an attack. Good martial arts practice does not generate fear of death or pain, and most students practice with enjoyment and confidence in their abilities and those of their partners to control their techniques. Nevertheless, the organism still has a natural, unconscious reaction upon observing a blow directed toward the eyes, but that stops a half inch from the face. Not only are the instincts of fight or flight activated by these actions, there is a moment in the soul where death is revealed as inevitable. The recovery from this state, and the effects of the unconscious reaction, are believed to be chemical, hormonal, and at the same time deeply spiritual. Even if the moment is short-lived, its effect causes essential changes to take place in the character of the individual. As these moments are repeated, the transformation becomes more pronounced and of longer duration. For many people it results in profound life-style changes.

The reinvention of the soul usually involves the stripping away of distractions and illusions to reveal a fundamental structure rather than an altering or rearranging of that structure. The survival of the organism still seems to rest upon the transmission of genetic code through millennia of evolutionary development, and our primal urges, instincts, and reactions are thought to be empowered by this. Martial arts study allows the practitioner to get in touch with these energies and influences, and in some cases confront and reconfigure them into a better-functioning balance. There is no question that one's true character is revealed in the *dojo*, both to others and as a mirror to oneself. The tradition and methodology allows for the pursuit of self-improvement, in the same progressive fashion as the improvement and perfection of technique. When students are able to put these psychological and spiritual concerns on the table with the physical, then they are truly engaged in a study of the Way, and all aspects of their lives become relevant to the inquiry.

To the outsider, the practice of martial arts merely appears more difficult as the training progresses. Technique seems more complicated, demands on the individual increase, and there are many more things to remember. While it also seems this way to beginning students much of the time, advanced students begin to see the path becoming clearer and simpler, the teachings fewer and more direct. It becomes apparent at some point (often around the black-belt level), that the more they know, the more they realize how much they do not know and how infinite that which is yet to be revealed may be. Only when this is accepted by students are they ready to study the real lessons of the martial arts, having acquired the basic physical, mental, and spiritual tools. Traditionally, this is the threshold of understanding that is represented by the black belt, and marks a new "beginning again" for students on their path up the mountain of mastery.

We see the principles of circularity and balance at work in the method of training, and the effect it has on those who practice martial arts with sincerity and willingness to learn. To most advanced students the simplicity of the traditions brings great joy and inspiration to their lives and practice. This knowledge becomes something they wish to share with others, and often they will annoy their friends along the way by extolling the virtues of the martial arts and encouraging them to join in. It is difficult to explain their fervor to those unfamiliar with this type of endeavor, or those who have been misled by common misconceptions about the martial arts. Unwilling to risk accusations of proselytizing or cult-like promotion, martial artists often console themselves with helping new students through their halting first steps in their own classes. This circulation of the energy between advanced and beginners enriches both their paths of study, and benefits the group as a whole. In schools where this interaction is systematically encouraged, the quality of the learning experience improves like a feedback loop. Students at intermediate levels are able to learn more, more quickly, and with greater understanding than those who went before. This helps keep their senior students honest, working hard, and not content to rest on their laurels. Over time, the individual and collective *kiai* becomes very strong because of this sharing of knowledge and encouragement.

A healthy *dojo*, like a healthy martial artist, is a living garden that requires nurturing, a sunny disposition, and occasional weeding. *Ki* energy can be seen as the energy of the water cycle, from rain to ground water and back again, through every vessel and cell, every inspiration, expiration, and transpiration of the organisms and elements present.

Martial artists are introduced to the reality of the universe in small steps, as they discover that by taking on more responsibility for themselves as individuals, their own health and fitness, spiritual serenity, and personal integrity, connection to others, and place in nature become revealed. Priorities become easier to assign and quality of life demands to be improved. By continuing with the training, through the steep slopes and periodic plateaus, the simple admonition to "breathe, relax, and smile," echoes in their ears and reminds them of the simple secrets of the martial arts.

Climbing to the Sky

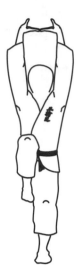

Stance: Stand with feet together and hands palm up, with fingertips touching in front of the abdomen.

Action: Shift the weight to the left foot, exhale, and slowly raise the right knee in front. Simultaneously bring both hands, palms up, from the abdomen to the face. Once the hands are at eye level, inhale and rotate them outward, palms down, thumbs toward the face. Continue to a palms-up, thumbs-up position reaching for the sky.

Exhale the air as you push the hands upward to their maximum reach. Bring the knee in toward your abdomen, keeping the support leg straight and hips horizontal.

Duration: Hold for a count of ten, then relax the position. Return by reversing the hands and knee motion. Repeat on the other side.

Comments: Maintain alignment and exhale from the abdomen. Avoid tilting neck and head backwards. Don't allow hip to slip to the side.

Catching the Star

Stance: Stand with feet shoulder width apart, and arms relaxed *(a)*.

Action: Inhale by expanding the abdomen. Open the arms slowly, turning the thumbs up and out and stretch the fingers to a maximum *(b)*. Once the arms are shoulder height and with the palms up, lift and stretch the toes *(c)*. Relax the toes and transfer the weight, then rise up on the balls of the feet, continuing with the full inhalation, until the hands reach high above the head. Feel the full elongation of the body, from the toes to the fingers *(d,* *e)*. Pause briefly in the breathing (without pressure). Place both hands palms together *(f)*. Follow with a slow exhalation of the air and controlled descent of the body until the heels touch the floor and the hands come together in front of the solar plexus *(g)*.

Repeat five cycles, with focus in the balance and on the breathing, trying to reach a farther star every time and storing it in the solar plexus energy center.

Rest between cycles in an envigorating and joyful way.

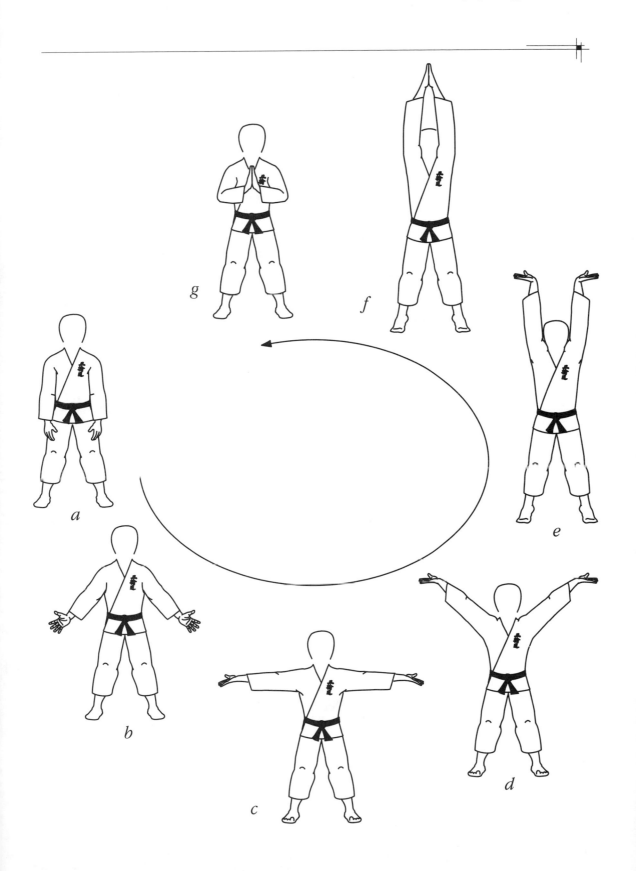

Secrets of the Martial Arts

- By summoning the internal energy of *ki*, focusing it with our mind, and releasing it with our spirit, we have created *kiai*.

- The real *kiai* is the union of energy itself; the shout its manifestation.

- When the student learns to coordinate the sound with the exhalation of air, then he begins to use *kiai* when strength or effort is required, as in lifting or striking.

- Board-breaking is not simply a trick to please crowds, but is useful in training *kime*, because in addition to the physical and mental, the spiritual dimension begins to enter the picture.

- The martial arts student is taught to *kiai* as the first response to a strike, hold, or grab. Most people think that the conditioning of this reflex is for the purpose of startling and distracting the attacker, and while it does serve this purpose, it is more important to help maintain breathing, strength levels, and to keep his wits together.

- When one is fatigued or exhausted, a few good *kiai* can awaken and revitalize oneself or a training partner.

- The *kiai* is a joyful noise unto the universe. In its pure form it connects the individual with his soul and that lonely soul with something greater.

- Transforming or redirecting anger, fear, and frustration into the joy of *kiai* allows the student to penetrate beyond the superficial and work toward a mastery of the self that is individual and enlightened.

- The opportunity to be reborn in the execution of a technique, or the deflection of an incoming attack, has a powerful effect on the attitude and spirit of the practitioner.

- One's true character is revealed in the *dojo*, both to others and as a mirror to oneself. The tradition and methodology allows for the pursuit of self-improvement, in the same progressive fashion as the improvement and perfection of technique.

Chapter 7

Stamina, Strength, and Speed

MARTIAL arts training is a specific approach to physical and mental development. Its method is based on a traditional line through which knowledge is passed from master to student. Within this framework, individual teachers in different circumstances will develop their own styles and ways of conducting their classes. Historically, these ways can diverge so greatly from traditional lines that their teachers can be said to have formed their own *ryu*, or school. Nevertheless, despite this branching of the family tree, we find general principles, specific techniques, philosophical underpinnings, and ceremonial traditions that have survived and flourished undiminished from the roots of this complex and varied system.

For most people, especially North Americans, physical education is an experience associated with their school years. Classes were typically conducted either by instructors who favored a military-style, calisthenics-based approach, or athletic coaches who organized sports such as football and basketball. Female phys-ed programs, if they existed, often had a gymnastics or folk dancing basis, with small doses of team sports like basketball or volleyball. These traditional teaching approaches were the natural result of having to deal with large groups of students, and were based on the knowledge and teaching experience available. There was also often pressure to live up to a reputation for sports prowess that was considered important for the image of the school and its alumni.

Although many skills and qualities can be developed through team sports and games, the process tended to benefit those who excelled, who made the team, especially the few who became star players. Many had natural talent for their game: the right body type, good reflexes, and proper attitude. Others overcame physical limitations such as size through determination and effort, becoming campus heroes in the process.

This glamorizing of sports figures carries into the present day and is magnified tremendously through the multi-billion dollar professional sports industry. Between Monday morning memories of back to school, and Monday night football on the couch, most people have been side-lined by the sports orientation of physical fitness. For these people, experiences in exercise classes are less than pleasant and often are reminders of inadequacy and failure. Simple running reduces some to exhaustion and tears. Mental revisitations of the class running around a gym or field, harassed by some guy with a whistle and a clipboard, are painful. Those who did not shine in these situations were less well served by the traditional phys-ed curriculum, which was designed to produce good teams and star athletes, not necessarily to develop the personal fitness of ordinary individuals.

Times have changed, and the education of exercise instructors has shifted focus. Schools of kinesiology and physical education are producing highly trained professionals to feed the profusion of health clubs, gyms, and fitness classes in community centers. Here, at least, winning isn't everything, but looking good sometimes seems to take precedence over staying fit and healthy. The social isolation of video-equipped machines and treadmills, at home or in a club, seems to fit perfectly with the urban segmentation of our lives. Even the group aerobics and step classes, with their loud music and mirrors, tends to distract us from ourselves rather than allowing us to embrace the body we have, work with it, and enjoy the sensation of physical exercise.

Martial arts training should be accessible to everyone. That doesn't mean necessarily that it *is* for everyone. Some are attracted to the martial arts for the wrong reasons and need to be turned away if their motives derive from aggressive or violent tendencies. Similarly, some-one who refuses to accept the discipline and traditions is wasting everyone's time, and should be shown the door for the sake of those who really want what the martial arts have to offer. With these elements addressed, anyone can participate, and should be able to attain excellence at their own level by applying themselves.

Many modern martial arts have adopted a colored belt system of marking a student's progress through the curriculum. In addition to systematizing what should be taught and in what order, the progression of belts allows students of various levels to work together in a single class. As we have mentioned, an important feature of martial arts is the role that senior students play in helping newer students along

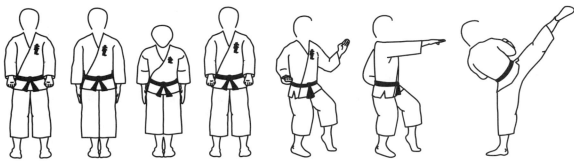

Opening movements of gorindo kata, called kiito nidan, including the bow which begins and ends every kata.

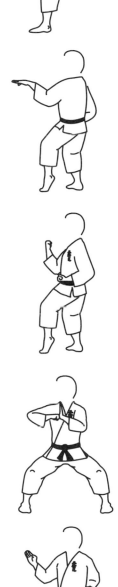

the path. The colors of sewn cotton should not be seen as achievement awards, but rather as indicators of what the student is ready to learn next. This important distinction discourages any idea that the recipient has fully mastered what has gone before. A fundamental precept of the training method is that the basics must be reviewed over and over, and that all skills will evolve as a result of realizations made at more advanced levels. This will be understood by beginners and seniors alike in a properly functioning *dojo* and is perhaps the most valuable contribution of the teaching methodology of the martial arts. This give and take, connecting as it does teacher and students, the principles of *nyuanshin*, and attention to good form, may also be the secret of the masters most easily abused or distorted by tournament competition, or the street fighting orientation of some modern schools.

Taoist and Confucian philosophies both emphasize that the long journey is made up of single steps. Zen philosophy as well focuses on the reality of the moment rather than the mountain peak up ahead. These concepts, so deeply rooted in the Asian mentality, are difficult for those of us raised in Western society to understand. Our goal-oriented, succeed-at-all-costs, to-the-winner-the-spoils mentality makes it difficult for us to appreciate achievement in those terms. Learning to enjoy the ride while still accomplishing excellent results is something that the martial arts can teach us.

How do the martial arts achieve this? How can they help improve our lives? The most direct answer is, by helping us get our priorities straight. Learning what is really important in our daily lives, how fragile the line between life and death, and how much can be accomplished if we chew manageable bites, are fundamentals of the training. From a health and fitness point of view, feeling well, enjoying balance and serenity, increasing longevity, and remaining active and engaged into a ripe old age count for much more than the quick fix for our "flab, abs, and butt." What can be quickly attained tends to be easily lost, and that is true of diet goals, muscle mass, and sculptured thighs, as well as other possessions.

But, what if we want more? For those already fit and healthy, but wanting to know the secrets of stamina, strength, and speed that lie in the training rituals of the martial arts, the keys to success are still the same: attention to basics, gradual progress, and practice, practice, practice. It is how the martial artist sets his mind, energy, and spirit to this task that sets him apart and gives him a completely different point of view regarding physical activity.

Size is never a true indication of muscular power and efficiency, as all Chinese boxing masters know only too well. The smaller man usually makes up for the balance of power by his greater agility, flexibility, speed of foot, and nervous action.

•

Bruce Lee

1940–73

The martial artist works cooperatively with himself, his body, his fellow students, and teacher. By submitting to the discipline and opening his life to examination, he can achieve much more. Many individual sports and exercise activities avoid tournaments, but nonetheless encourage participants to compete with themselves. As well, many teachers claim that "the only enemy is yourself," but what is the value of this? Why fight when you could be friends? What kind of life is it when you speak, eat, and sleep with the enemy? How can this lead to happiness?

Training in a cooperative, friendly environment, where you respect your partner and treat him well so that he can return to train with you the next day, is essential in the martial arts. Even though the actual techniques involve smashing and punching and over-throwing of your partner, the goal is learning, not winning, and the environment that is conducive to learning is one that must be cultivated by principle, effort, and diligence. These are attributes that will then be available at anytime and anywhere during the whole of one's life. Here, we see that the martial arts are undeniably physical, but are fueled by the mental and spiritual processes that inform, and are a result of, the training.

A successful exercise program based on the martial arts has several requirements, and these apply equally to a single-class session and the program as a whole. It begins with a good warm-up, starting slowly and simply then gradually accelerating; it has a variety of activities to maintain interest; it reinforces important health objectives, such as sleeping and eating well, managing stress, remaining limber, active and able; it utilizes the left and right sides of the brain and body, in balance;

it operates on all planes of movement; and it has respect for individual learning curves and ranges of physical development.

Training with these principles in the martial arts will allow all types of people to do things they have never done before, to endure and excel, even under unusual conditions, to reveal and discover their true character, and to define and focus their lives. All of this flows from the practice because it provides students with basic tools and a workshop to build in.

So, how does martial arts training turn a beginner into a black belt? Let's look at an individual class. After the introductory formalities and a brief meditation, students prepare themselves with a standard warm-up. Often senior students will take turns conducting this portion of the class, as it gives them an opportunity to practice their vocal and observational skills, and the other students become accustomed to their voices and teaching styles, rather than focusing on the *sensei* all the time.

The first elements taught are the foundation stances. Correct foot position, distribution of weight, and balanced alignment are established, and then, depending on group size and space available, the students will learn to move forward and backward, taking repetitive steps. Basic hand movements are then incorporated, usually simple blocks and punches, and attention is paid to relaxed shoulders, exhalation during execution, and avoiding hypertension of the joints, particularly the elbow and knee.

While the beginners are struggling with distinguishing left from right, the length of their stances, and keeping up with the line, the intermediate and advanced students have their own work cut out for them. They will sometimes be given additional combinations of strikes or kicks, to be completed within the same stepping movement or timing count. In *aikido* and *judo*, entrances, half steps, and segments of techniques are repetitively practiced as *kihon*, basics. Advanced students use this time to incorporate something new they are working on, in breathing, mental state, or technique, or possibly some simple correction of the big toe, elbow position, or facial grimace, that has been pointed out to them in practice. The most advanced students will still be struggling with the same priorities as the beginner: relaxed shoulders, correct position, and alignment and balance, although hopefully with more consistent success, and usually in a way that is almost invisible to observers, unless they are experienced teachers.

Few other activities place such conscious emphasis on reworking the basics as do the martial arts. It can sometimes be

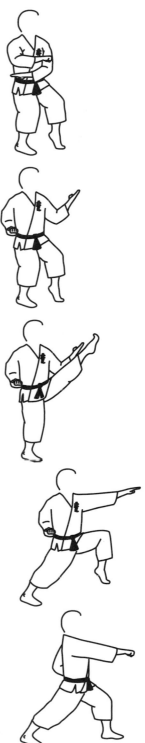

When well-executed, a movement can have the natural power of a wave crashing on the shore.

Examples of Gorindo Kihon

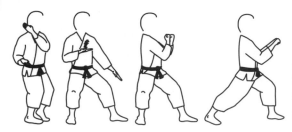

Movements practice shifting of the weight in a change of stance, use of open hands and both arms simultaneously, and acquiring a sense of body width.

Other movements focus on balance and chamber training, use of the double kick with change of height, and controlled landing in back stance with upper body defense.

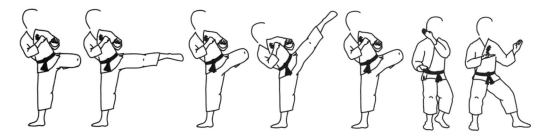

frustrating for beginners as they develop some proficiency, to find themselves practicing the same skills they learned on the first day. Usually their reaction is: "I know that one already, let's move on to something new." It is the skilled teacher who can lead students through repetitive practice in ways that keeps students interested, involved, and still learning. Basics must be identified clearly as foundation building blocks, not just simplified versions of techniques meant for beginners alone. At the same time, glimpses of the complex and inviting things to come must be revealed without the student feeling that secrets are being kept from him.

Kihon then, is the main engine of the martial arts learning process. New techniques that have been introduced by demonstration and explanation are incorporated into the learned mental and physical vocabulary. They are refined through practice while moving backward, forward, sideways, inside out, and with different speed and intensity. New twists are added to keep students on their toes, and while the mind is engaged with learning, the body is increasing aerobic capacity, cardiopulmonary efficiency, and overall flexibility and strength.

Maintaining balance and learning to turn quickly, to the dominant as well as the less used side, is important in these exercises. As the

Balance while using the hands in different trajectory and planes, and simultaneous defense and counterattack skills are developed.

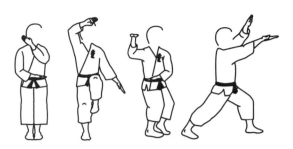

Perception of backward and 360° turns, control of the hips, and landing with equal distribution of body weight are practiced as well.

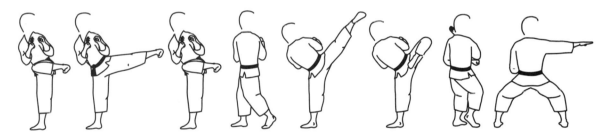

students identify with the counting, especially in an unfamiliar language, they find a rhythm to their movements that helps relax the breathing, and frees the mind from directing the coordination of arms and legs. Once the pattern has been acquired, the student must learn not to think about the individual movements, and instead, let the combination flow as one movement. A good rhythm can help unite the group in these efforts, and a collective energy or "groove" can be developed, much in the same way as a group of musicians learns to breathe and play together. This synergistic energy can encourage weaker, slower, or more tired members to carry on in step with their fellow trainees. This should not be confused with a competitive approach to be faster, more dynamic, or to kick higher than the person on either side. The student should be encouraged to achieve a synchronicity of movement with the group, by being in time with the others, mentally present, and giving maximum effort. By uniting according the principle that the whole is greater than the sum of its parts, everyone can tap into a source of energy that can be tangibly felt. Although it is difficult to measure scientifically, this goodwill and intensity can allow the individual student to overcome feelings of fatigue, frustration, or inadequacy, and thus reach performance levels beyond previously perceived limits. Once this

An example of an ippon kumite *combination showing recognition, reaction, movement, redirect, and control, with the collaboration of a partner.*

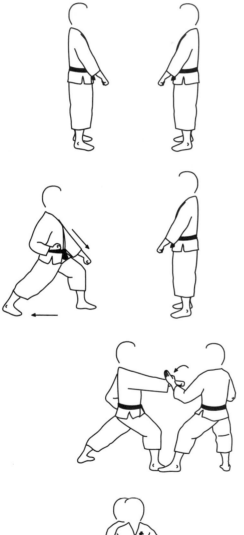

ability has been revealed in the group context it is easier to utilize the lessons for individual development of personal resources.

With attention to the changing demands of the cardiovascular system and monitoring and controlling the breathing dynamic during *kihon*, energy levels in the body can be maintained and improved. The use of the *kiai* can relax the abdomen, ensure the exhalation of waste carbon dioxide, focus the technique for maximum efficiency, and stimulate the energy of students. Collective *kiai* can also make the room vibrate and encourages strong joyful spirit.

Kihon relies on repetition to achieve numerous goals. Practice is practice, and some physical and mental processes require numerous "firings" in the same pattern to create pathways in the brain and body that can then be accessed reflexively. Good hard practice of technique that is correct and balanced allows stamina and strength to build readily without damage or strain.

Repetition also allows muscles to be warmed, joints lubricated, and oxygen to flow freely. Tense muscles become loose, and as they tire other muscles take up the slack. These "secondary" muscles often are not exercised until this changing of shift occurs. As they become strong, a better balance is achieved within muscle groupings, which improves the overall technique and fitness of the practitioner. Once the body and mind are conditioned for these movements, speed and power can be developed. Development of explosive movement

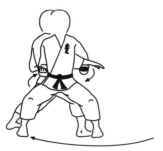
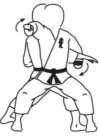
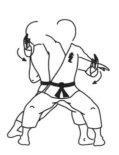
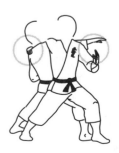

and work with resistance, impact, and weight are advanced stages of this progression, undertaken only when the body is fully prepared.

Repetition of a known combination allows the mind to be concerned with the essentials of the technique, the accuracy of placement, the movement of the target, and the changing of energy. In martial arts the mind should be fully engaged *in* the technique rather than dwelling *on* the technique. This state of mind is quite different from other repetitive exercise such as aerobics, running, and swimming. There the mind is encouraged to become detached and wander, to avoid monotony while allowing feelings of euphoria, excitement, or other emotions to color the experience. Many people participate in these activities to escape, problem solve, or just think about things. There is nothing inherently wrong with this, and many martial artists enjoy such activities for the same reasons, but they approach their own training with a different purpose. The demand for absolute attention in order to avoid injury, the philosophical principles behind the discipline, and the reality of the self-defense underpinnings of martial arts, mitigate against this kind of "spaced-out" participation. Without the mental aspect, even with health and fitness goals as the priority, much that is valuable and special in martial arts can be lost or go unrealized.

Good practice allows the student to eliminate errors of technique in the early stages. Foot position and alignment of the spine are critical in preventing injuries, both in the short and long term. It is in *kihon* that the student develops a feel for natural movement that serves him well when it comes to *kata* or *kumite* and advanced technique. When the body is moving in a natural or balanced way, the movement seems as if it is happening to you rather than you having to do it or force effort into the technique. Again, many musicians will tell you that with the right circumstances, one merely "falls into the groove," and playing can seem effortless and inspired during those times. Martial artists aspire to that kind of flow in their practice and, by extension, in their entire lives.

The desire for self-improvement in all areas of physical and mental capacity is central to the training goals. Acquiring stamina and strength is all in aid of being able to move and think with more ease, efficiency,

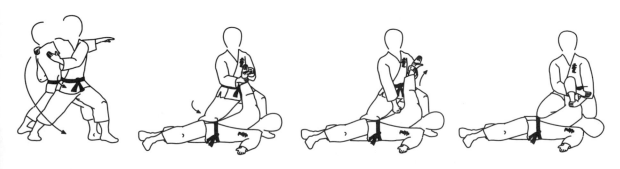

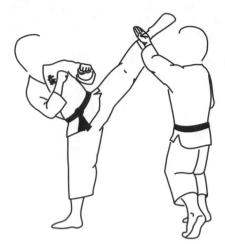

There is a great beauty in the control, rhythm, agility, and accuracy of the movements of jiyu kumite.

and pleasure. Although there is no question that true martial art training is rigorous and at times difficult, one of the secrets of why it works so well is the relationship of effort and efficiency. The hard work has to be oriented toward a productive goal, and not just exist because tradition dictates that the training be demanding. Too much sweat and fatigue, in fact, can often mean that tension is being carried in the body; they do not necessarily mean that one is obtaining an optimum workout. The effort may be there, but not the results. Sweat should be the consequence of good intensity and as the workout progresses, relaxation should increase. This can create a paradox for the advanced student because as technique improves things should get "easier." While it is true that the same technique will be smoother and more efficient, drawing less effort from the body, the capability to do more is increased, allowing the advanced student to perform with more focus and intensity. The martial artist must practice *nyuanshin* to continue to flourish at advanced levels.

In order to develop speed, the use of tension and relaxation needs to be coordinated. Students practice confining tension to those areas that require it—explosive propulsion, jumping, or the launching of a technique—while the rest of the body remains relaxed. Being able to take advantage of gravity, centrifugal and centripetal forces for unbalancing and circular techniques, requires relaxation in the limbs and limberness in the shoulders and hips.

In the language of the physicist, the kinetic energy delivered by a technique is a function of mass and velocity (KE= $\frac{1}{2}$ mv²), but as laymen, let us think weight and speed. Speed is more important in the actual equation because, as you can see, it multiplies itself; a small increase in speed will thus have a much greater effect on the power exerted than the mass of the weapon used. This allows a smaller person to increase the power of his strike or kick without increasing his size or weight (not realistic possibilities in any case). In the same way that a fragile straw can be driven into the trunk of a tree by the force

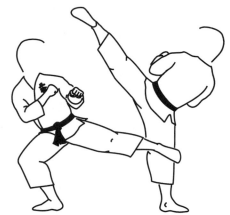

Good kumite *is a conversation between two partners.*

of a hurricane, speed and accurate technique can become an powerful combination.

Although we might assume that a larger person is still more powerful than a smaller person with equivalent technique, we must also consider that the smaller person has a lower center of gravity, a smaller target area, and possibly the element of surprise as countervailing advantages. We have mentioned how the person with dominant upper body strength tends to use that strength rather than hip action. Mobility also, can be limited by high center of gravity and tension across the chest and shoulders. The massive person, especially the weight-lifting type, is often slower, less flexible, and top heavy. The person accustomed to using size for intimidation, and brute force to make his way in the world, may thus easily be defeated by the smaller martial artist who uses these advantages of his size. Confronting a variety of training partners in the *dojo* allows students to learn their own strengths and weaknesses, and how those will interact with others of different size and experience.

Kihon is practiced to develop technique, coordination, and stamina, and is a variable and directed activity. At an early stage in the training, a different type of exercise is introduced that serves the same purposes and many additional ones. *Kata* is a formalized, controlled, dance-like pattern with visualized partners. It literally means "the optimal form" or "the correct way" and is accorded huge respect in the traditional Japanese arts. Its importance extends beyond the merely apparent, because of the mental and spiritual requirements that must combine with the physical in order for *kata* to be performed well. For many, the *kata* is the ultimate expression of the "art" in martial art.

Kata is learned initially as a method of acquiring coordination and fluidity in executing combinations, but eventually *kata* becomes a meditation in motion for the body and the mind. It is the code for deciphering the many variations and combinations of technique available; the key to unlocking reserves of energy and spiritual awakenings; the resting place for the mind, body, and spirit in times of confusion and stress; and finally a dance of grace, virtue, and strength that celebrates the joy of martial arts training. By putting it all together in the *kata*, maximum effort is expended, maximum focus is required, and maximum benefit obtained. The practice of well-designed and well-executed *kata* is a fundamental secret of martial art.

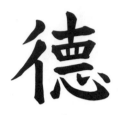

Toku:
virtue, or power

Every movement is planned in the *kata*, including the movement of the eyes and the breath. While perfection is sought, as in the cutting and polishing of a fine diamond, it is never thought to have been achieved. There should always be room for a better execution of a *kata*. It is exact and should not be varied, yet in the precise framework that is defined for movement *kata* feels very expressive to the practitioner. As the body and mind are united in the performance of the prescribed techniques, the spirit is freed from decision over *what* should be done *next*, and more involved in *how* it should be done *now*.

Each *kata* begins and ends with a formal bow, reminding the practitioner to focus on the *kata*, be composed in the moment, and pay respect to the spirit of the *kata* and the *sensei* by doing it well. With its distinct beginning and end, the student has the opportunity to create an absolutely new performance, free from the errors or weaknesses of the past.

Kata are not usually easy to learn; they require positions that challenge the balance, equilibrium, and coordination. They provide confidence and internalization of technique. As a benchmark for the contemplation of progress, and the analysis of improvements and changes, they are useful intellectual tools, offering interesting realizations about character, feelings, and emotions. When body, mind, and spirit can be brought into balance, a meditative state of high performance can be achieved and explored. This is a state that can be accessed at other times, when there are more variables, and more order, focus, or energy is needed.

Kata are often quite beautiful, and when fully imbued with a pure *kiai*, can be devastatingly powerful. Although the modern competitive approach to *kata* as dance or theater, with music, costumes, and props can be very entertaining, a simple traditional *kata* performed correctly and honestly will carry resonance that echoes in time.

There is no end to the practice of *kata*. Its repetitions, unlike those of the *kihon*, are of a longer period and therefore never feel routine. *Kata* practice alone, once a good level of technique has been achieved, can provide a complete workout in terms of cardiovascular conditioning, strength and flexibility, and when repeated a thousand times, which is the traditional minimum, improves stamina, patience, and character.

Practicing *kata* well can benefit all other aspects of martial arts training, even when practiced alone. Those who must be absent from working with partners due to travel, work, or family obligations still find that by continuing the practice of the *kata* on their own, their fitness, reflexes, and flexibility are maintained and they can return to the full training relaxed and strong.

There is a tendency among some in the martial arts to eschew *kata* training because of a mistaken belief that time would be better spent just sparring or practice fighting. However, most well-rounded martial artists know that their skills in this area are improved by faithful *kata* practice, even when there has been no practice of sparring. Reflexes, timing, and stamina will still improve with *kata*. It cannot, however, be said that the reverse is true.

Sparring, or *kumite*, like *kata* and *kihon* is a component of martial arts training. It should be viewed as an opportunity to react to new situations and to act intuitively. It is an exercise in training the reactions to allow a coordinated mind and body to neutralize attacks with appropriate technique. Good technique must be fast, with timing and flow and without hesitation or deliberation, both responding to, and redirecting the intentions and actions of the opponent. *Kumite* is an exchange, a communication between two persons, not just attacking and blocking, kicking, and punching. *Kata* and *kumite* have been described as the sun and the moon of martial arts practice.

Many animals in nature engage in play fighting. Often an adult will teach skills to an infant, or young ones will just roughhouse with each other. Large animals will get down on their knees to play with smaller partners. Some psychological studies have postulated that this activity is an essential part of healthy touching and is fundamental to a balanced personality.

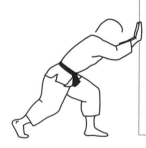

THE role of the *daisansha* in *gorindo kumite* practice is to observe interactively, guard the health and safety of the participants, and ensure a friendly discipline, as a third party to the exchange.

RULES OF *GORINDO* CONTACT PRACTICE:
1. NO ONE GETS HURT.
2. NO ONE HURTS ANYBODY.
3. REMEMBER RULES 1 AND 2.
4. HAVE FUN.
5. BREATHE, RELAX, AND SMILE.

When *kumite* is regarded as an improving experience, rather than a testing one, it is easier to give and receive blows with a positive attitude. Although a basic component of martial arts is self-defense, one partner has to consent to an attacking role, so that the other can practice defense and countermovement. Unfortunately, the common presentation of sparring for points, trophies, and medals rewards only the attack, and not a brilliant defense. More critically, it does not recognize the skill of not fighting at all. True *kumite* practice, as opposed to sparring or fighting, must be playful, inspired, and joyful, without hurting your partner emotionally, physically, or spiritually.

Kumite, once unburdened by competitive baggage, can be thought of as a discourse between friends, and a good session will make you want to hug your partner at the end. When good *kumite* is watched on film or video without a sound track, one can more easily see the mutual exchange of energy and the moves become complementary rather than opposing. When participating in *kumite* one should aspire to the same calm mental state that is practiced in meditation and *kata*.

Kata has a plan, while *kumite* has no plan. *Kata* is formality in a pure sense and *kumite* transmits free movement and expression. *Ippon kumite* (one-step, pre-arranged sparring) introduces the element of choice in response to opposing movement. Techniques become more complex in a progressive fashion, leading to the rhythms and reactions of the "free sparring," or *jiyu kumite*.

The Sun and Moon of Martial Arts Practice

KATA	KUMITE
ordered	spontaneity
reason	passion
structured	formless
empty / full	giving / taking
independence	co-dependance
here	now
index of technique	improvised technique
responsibility for oneself	responsibility for another
creativity	adaptation
flexibility	stability
has a map	has no map
adapts to shape of the container	creates the shape of the container

Kumite raises the emotions and instincts to the surface from a deeper, unconscious level. In the context of martial arts training, this requires that the student have a good understanding of the purpose of the exercise, and how it needs to be integrated into both his physical and attitudinal responses. The level of excited awareness and the effects of even accidental contact heighten the likelihood of minor injury. This is another reason that *kumite* should only be practiced by more advanced students. *Kumite* should only be introduced when the student has acquired proficiency of movement, and the ability to block and maintain a good guard. Many students have become discouraged with martial arts training when asked to spar too soon. Schools that depend on tournament participation for promotion and financial support can be pushing their students into situations that they are unprepared for, both physically and mentally. When properly integrated into a balanced martial arts curriculum, *kumite* offers unique practice opportunities and learning situations. The mental focus, and expansion of spirit and character, are just as important as the physical requirements for successful *kumite*. In a school where training partners can engage in this type of exchange safely and harmoniously, great strides can be made in the development of technique, physique, and intelligence.

Because *kumite* involves an equally vulnerable human body offering itself as a moving target, the demand for control, caution, and compassion are at the highest levels. Even the extreme forms of full-contact engagement still have rules and limitations to protect the combatants. *Kumite*, whether of the striking, throwing, or grappling kind, exercises strength and stamina, but still must be carefully constrained. When strength can be exercised so as to be subtle and sensitive, and yet flows with speed and accuracy, a martial art is being practiced, not fighting. Brute force can be effectively neutralized by intelligent application of the laws of physics, dynamic energy, and sometimes the ability to just roll with the punches.

The highly polished technique, seamless coordination of fine and gross motor skills, and conditioned physiological responses of the advanced martial artist, are a result of the combined knowledge of hundreds of years of practice and study. In order that the harnessing of such power can be brought about for purposes of peaceful co-existence and the goals of health and fitness, a philosophical mindset must be maintained. The teaching method prepares the body, mind, and character for the responsibilities and rewards of being a martial artist. Although not everyone wishes to train at the level of expertise the advanced forms of martial art training demands, every student should be prepared to accept that they are working toward that ability and respect the traditions which shape that progress.

Seiza and Yoko-geri, Side Kick

Stance: *Seiza*, kneeling position, sitting on the heels with the torso vertical.

Action: Reach forward and place both palms on the floor in front of you with hands directly under shoulders. With spine straight and arms extended, bring the left knee up to the side just behind the left shoulder. Then push and extend the leg in a side-kick motion (leading with the outside edge of the heel while flexing the ankle). Return the knee to the shoulder level before lowering it to the ground. Repeat five times on each side.

Comments: Remember that the higher the kick the lower the chest should be, with more body weight on the arms. Bend the elbows slightly. Be aware of the transfer from four to three points of support and balance. Exhale when kicking. and *kiai*.

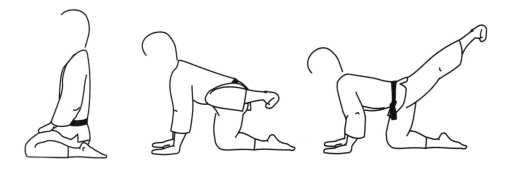

Sensei Uensei Stretch

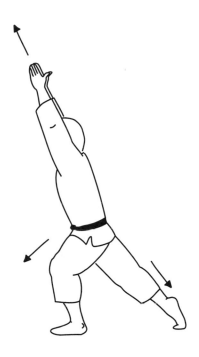 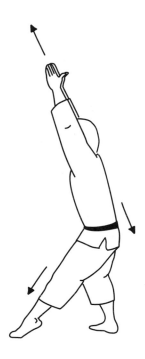

Stance: Left foot forward the distance of a walking step, hands and arms together reaching toward the sky, legs straight.

Action: Flex the front knee and raise the back heel. Exhale and feel the length of the body as if it is stretching from the fingers into the sky and the rear leg into the earth. Return and inhale. Next phase, bring the rear heel to the floor and shift the weight to the right leg, straightening the left leg and pointing the toes, keeping the upper body the same. Exhale and hold the stance. Repeat five times on each side. This exercise stretches and strengthens the legs, back, torso and upper body. This motion can be adapted to a self-defense maneuver that relies on extension and displacement.

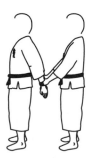 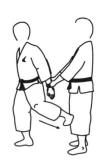 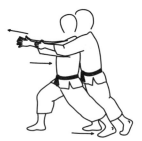 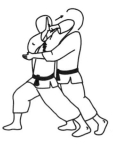 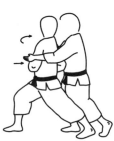

Gorindo Kihon
First Basic Series

The purpose of the basic series is to acquaint the beginning student with how to stand, how to protect different regions of the body, how to coordinate left and right hands, and to breathe comfortably with *kiai* (union of energy) in the techniques. It is a repetitive exercise practiced in a stationary location using basic stances, strikes, and blocks. It should be performed slowly at first with the emphasis on correct and complete technique. As coordination and body awareness improve, the pace can be increased, but a smooth energetic rhythm should be maintained. As the series becomes more familiar, the focus of attention shifts to awareness of the center of gravity, the center line of the body, and the dimensions of the body in different planes. In the class situation the student may practice individually, in mirror image with a partner, or as a synchronized group.

While doing the series, let your eyes contemplate the area in front of you in a relaxed manner, as if you are watching a big movie screen. Avoid focusing on the height of the technique. Check your posture, keeping the pelvis underneath you and knees slightly bent.

Pay attention to the breathing rhythm. Take time to ensure technique is accurate, then progressively increase speed. The breathing pattern will change from one breath per strike or block to a longer period that flows over several repetitions.

Exercise Sequence

Practice each sequence of punches and blocks in each of the stances below.
Return to standing position after each change of stance.

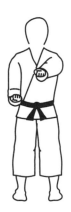 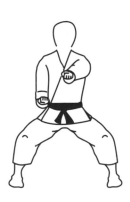 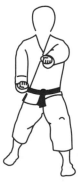 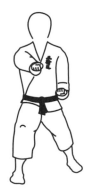

Heiko-dachi
Ready stance

Hiba-dachi
Horse-riding stance

Hidari zenkutsu-dachi
Left front stance

Migi zenkutsu-dachi
Right front stance

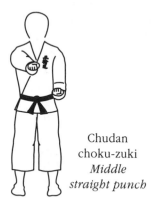

Chudan
choku-zuki
*Middle
straight punch*

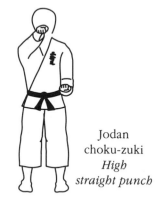

Jodan
choku-zuki
*High
straight punch*

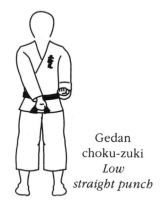

Gedan
choku-zuki
*Low
straight punch*

Practice the alternating punches (left and right)
with ten strikes to each region: middle, high and low.
Kiai after each round of ten.

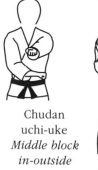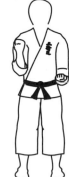

Chudan
uchi-uke
*Middle block
in-outside*

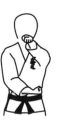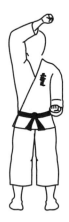

Jodan
age-uke
High block

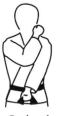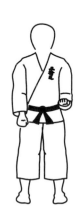

Gedan-barai
Low block

Practice the alternating defenses (left and right)
with ten blocks to each region: middle, high and low.
Kiai after each round of ten.

Gorindo Kata Geometrica
Triangle, Circle, and Square

This series of exercises should be practiced as a group. It can be thought of as a stationary *kata*, involving as it does a progression of movements that strengthens, stretches, and loosens almost every area of the body. From these three shapes, which operate on three planes of movement, other shapes and vectors can be drawn. Emphasis is on smooth movement, balance, and focused breathing using the abdomen. Move as if the imaginary ball you hold is a bowl filled with precious elixir and you do not want to spill a drop. Position of stances, pelvis, and head are very important. Hand movements are precise and very controlled but with shoulders, elbows, and fingers remaining relaxed.

It is important as a mental exercise to visualize the geometric shape the hands are creating as they move through the form. As well, the body with its stance and shifting of weight should feel as if it is describing the triangle, circle, or square.

By leading with the eyes and co-ordinating the breathing with the movement, a smooth flow can be established. Feel as if you are breathing through your hands. Pay close attention to the perimeters of hand and knee movements to not place undue stress or extension on the joints. Observe the diagram and practice in front of mirror or glass reflection initially to check position.

Practice synchronizing the movements with the breathing, seeking to elongate the exhalation.

Gorindo Triangle

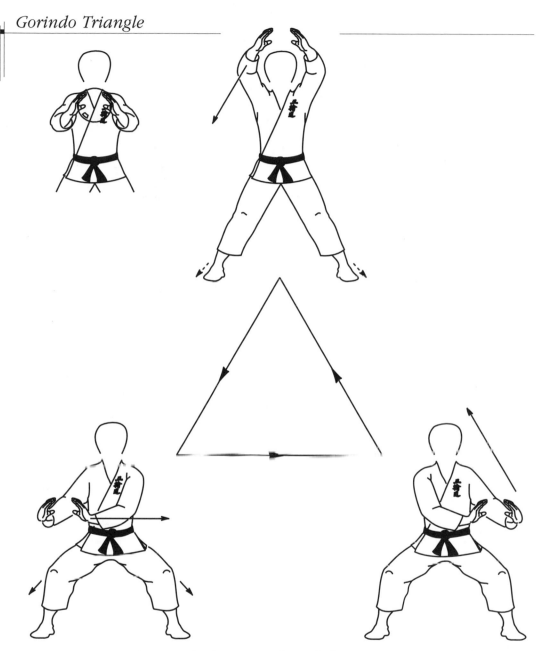

Stance: Approximately triangular, heels slightly inside with feet flat on floor. Weight remains equally distributed, without shifting, throughout exercise.

Action: Begin by forming imaginary ball (volleyball size) in your mind and place it within your hands in front of chest. Lift ball above your head with a gentle intake of breath. Exhale in a controlled fashion through nose as you bend your knees and lower ball to the right side. Completely empty lungs by contracting abdomen muscles as you move the ball across the body from right to left. Let the lungs inflate as you raise hands and body to standing position. Relax abdomen and throat as air enters the nose and partially open mouth. Rest at top of motion.

Repeat four times and then perform four triangles in the opposite direction.

Gorindo Circle

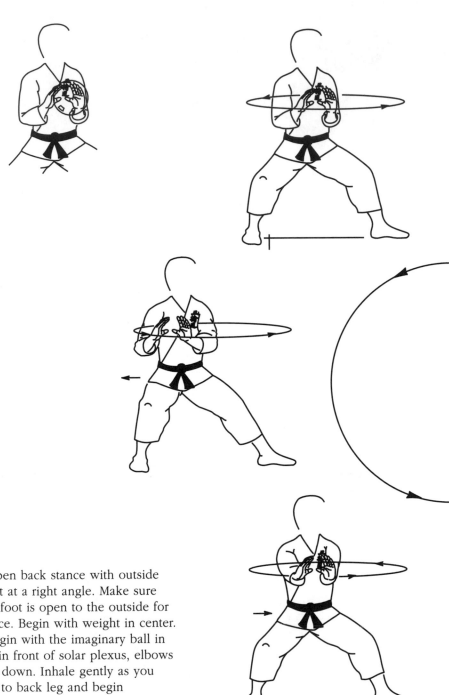

Stance: Open back stance with outside edges of feet at a right angle. Make sure the forward foot is open to the outside for stable balance. Begin with weight in center.

Action: Begin with the imaginary ball in your hands in front of solar plexus, elbows relaxed and down. Inhale gently as you shift weight to back leg and begin describing circle with hands to the outside and back. Begin to exhale as you push

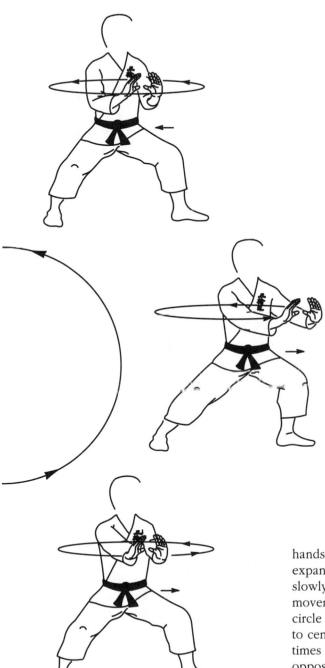

hands forward and away from you to expand the circle outward. Shift the weight slowly to the forward leg along with the movement of the hands. Complete the circle by bringing hands and hips back to center. Rest for a moment. Repeat four times and then perform four circles in the opposite direction, placing other foot forward in the stance.

Gorindo Square Up

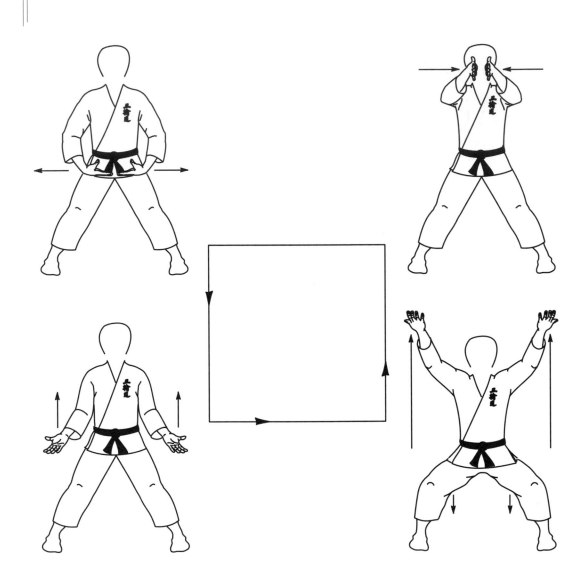

Stance: Square horse-riding stance. Stand with outside edges of feet parallel and two shoulder widths apart.

Action: Begin with fingers touching, palms up, below *hara*. Inhale gently as the hands move outward. Rotate fingers forward and raise palms toward the sky while bending knees. Keep buttocks tucked in and exhale as the body lowers. Exhale fully, emptying lungs completely as you rise to a standing position while pressing hands together in front of face. Inhale as the hands drop to *hara* position. Repeat four times.

Gorindo Square Down

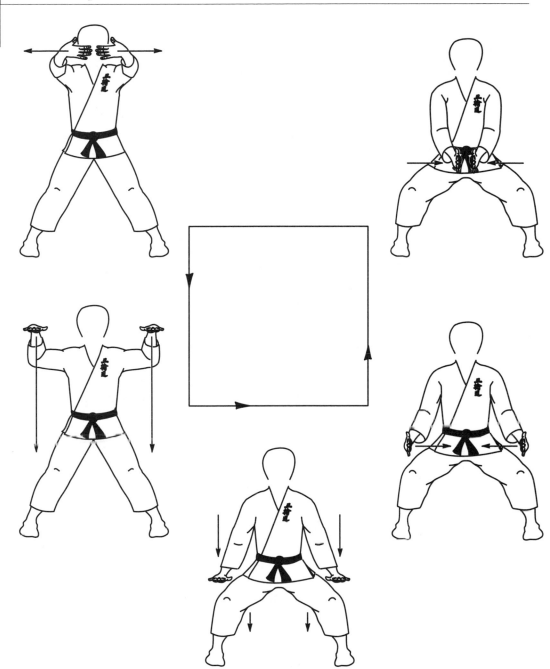

Stance: Square horse-riding stance. Stand with outside edges of feet parallel and two shoulder widths apart.

Action: Begin with hands in front of the face, pulling apart as you inhale gently. Press downward with hands, exhaling as you lower body and emptying lungs completely as the hands are pushed together again in front of *hara*. Inhale as you raise hands and body to start position. Repeat four times.

Secrets of the Martial Arts

- The secrets of building stamina, strength, and speed in martial arts training are simply: attention to basics, gradual progress, and practice, practice, practice.

- Basics, or *kihon*, must be identified clearly as foundation building blocks, not just simplified versions of techniques meant for beginners alone.

- The student should be encouraged to achieve a synchronicity of movement with the group, by being present, on time, and giving maximum effort.

- Once the body and mind are conditioned to perform *kata* movements, then speed and power can be developed. Development of explosive movement and work with resistance, impact, and weight are advanced stages of this progression, when the body is fully prepared.

- Excess sweat and fatigue can often mean that there is tension in the body, and not necessarily that one is obtaining an optimum workout.

- In order to develop speed, the use of tension and relaxation must be coordinated. Students practice confining tension to those areas that require it.

- *Kata* is a formalized, controlled, dance-like pattern with visualized partners. It literally means "the optimal form" or "the correct way" and is accorded huge respect in the traditional Japanese arts.

- *Kata* practice alone, once a good level of technique has been achieved, can provide a complete workout in terms of cardiovascular conditioning, stamina, strength, and flexibility.

- *Kumite* should be an exchange, a communication between two persons, not just attacking and blocking, kicking, and punching. *Kata* and *kumite* have been described as the sun and the moon of martial arts practice.

- True *kumite* practice, as opposed to sparring or fighting, must be playful, inspired, and joyful, without hurting your partner, emotionally, physically, or spiritually.

Chapter 8

What is Self-defense?

MANY people become involved in the martial arts because they wish to learn how to defend themselves. Quite naturally, they presume that they will learn to punch, kick, and overthrow their opponent, but do they really know what they are preparing to defend themselves against? Although we all share to some degree a primeval fear of the dark, it is more likely that our fear of alleys and parking lots comes from the dark corners of prime-time TV. Still, although the risk of attack from a mugger or rapist on the street is very small, it is nevertheless real.

Short courses for women in self-defense, and anti-rape devices such as pepper spray and shrieking horns are popular, but opinion varies on their usefulness. Although old-fashioned ideas about submitting to rape to avoid further injury are generally rejected, even trained martial artists agree that it is not worth fighting an armed attacker over a wallet or watch. Clearly the rules of engagement are not simple and the meaning of self-defense is more complicated than it at first appears.

Let us begin, then, with an understanding of what we are trying to protect. Every man, woman, and child has the right to personal liberty, privacy, and autonomy. We adjust these rights within the reasonable limits imposed by our need to gather in social groups. Although we traditionally come together to accomplish certain shared goals, on a personal level we all wish to go about our business without hindrance; we want to eat, sleep, work, spend good times with family and friends, and limit our exposure to fear, pain, and violence. This utopian vision, is in fact, a fairly accurate portrait how most of us do spend our lives in modern, wealthy democracies. Although different cultures view the

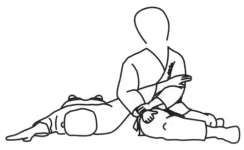

The practice of defensive breaks and restraining holds can actually massage pressure points and loosen joints.

necessity of the telephone, hot and cold running water, and the two-car garage quite differently, our basic needs as humans for health and happiness are fundamentally the same. Ultimately, it is not our possessions but our health and happiness that we wish to protect from harm.

Martial artists practice the art of self-defense in all its conventional aspects, but go further in using the same principles to avoid and deflect attacks on their physical, mental, and spiritual well-being. Improved awareness, good powers of observation, quick reflexes, and precise evasive movements will all come in handy in other areas of our lives. Just stepping off the curb to cross a street as a distracted or aggressive driver careens around the corner, presents a dangerous situation. The skills and faculties developed through martial arts training can help us escape. Stress reduction and anger management through relaxation and meditation will limit the chances of heart disease, stroke, and cancer, and generally make life calmer and more pleasant. Strengthened spiritual fortitude and a well-developed sense of self allow us to deal with the emotions involved when misfortune does strike, and can be one of the most valuable benefits of martial arts training as well.

Broadening the scope of self-defense into one that is more personal and truly of the "self" helps to build a framework for both the ethical and practical aspects of the pursuit of the martial arts. One must remember that the traditions and history of martial arts range from the peaceful Shaolin monks, who learned to defend themselves when their vows would not allow the use of weapons, through the samurai who seemed to be rising constantly, sword in hand, to some challenge to their personal honor or that of their master, to the present day spiritual warrior who pursues the ancient art of *tai chi chuan* in a park.

Many people have been deterred from the practice of martial arts simply because they don't want to hurt anybody. Probably equal in numbers are those who don't wish to get injured themselves, and are uncertain of how potentially lethal techniques can be learned without someone being hurt. However, as we have seen, it is precisely because of the respect, traditions, and attention to consistant progressive prac-

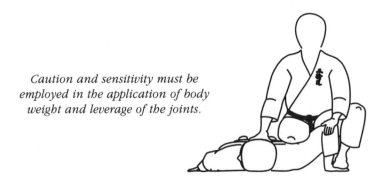

Caution and sensitivity must be employed in the application of body weight and leverage of the joints.

tice, that the long-term study of martial arts can offer a safe, effective approach to self-defense.

Although learning a few techniques in a seminar or a magazine article may in fact save someone's life, the benefits of these experiences should not be confused with the rewards of a serious study of martial arts. The difference between a woman who has just learned the eye poke, throat jab, or the traditional knee to the groin, and a woman practicing at an advanced level in a well-rounded martial arts school, is the degree of freedom from fear she experiences when walking down the street. The well-trained martial artist will still exercise caution and vigilance in her daily life, and not entertain illusions about being invulnerable to attack. However, she knows that if such a rare attack occurs, she possesses a range of well-practiced options, from escape to complete immobilization of the assailant. Depending upon the situation, she might even use her training to stay calm and talk her way out of immediate danger. The point is that her training allows her choices, including non-lethal restraining techniques, whereas the novice has no recourse but to the single, radical technique she has been taught.

Obviously, it is not only women who are subject to violence and experience the immobilizing fear of attack. Many men join martial arts schools to learn self-defense, but for some reason are less willing to admit that motivation to others.

People with little training who find themselves in violent situations are often frozen by the enormity of having their worst fears realized, and this is compounded by the awful realization that they might have to kill someone to escape. The long-term effects of the violence on the psyche of those who survive such attacks can sometimes be worse than any physical damage.

Fear and anger are the worst enemies of the martial artist. That is why the training must address these issues by preparing students to recognize, accept, and overcome them. Confidence and serenity come from having a healthy strong body, trained reflexes, and experience in meeting an attack. The martial artist claims the right to walk without disabling fear and yet still exercises caution. The student leaves the *dojo* armed with technique, spirit, and a well-balanced character that knows its limitations.

Many people consider martial arts training after they have been attacked or made to fear for their safety or that of their families. They might, for example, enter a short course of self-defense and think that they have studied martial art. They have learned a few techniques, but they have not really been empowered. What they truly require to live comfortably within their environment, is the power that comes from feeling healthy and strong. This gives them confidence in their own abilities, belief in their fundamental right to exist in the universe without hindrance, and the mental stability to shake off dark imaginings.

The purpose of striking and kicking in practice becomes not an attempt to destroy an enemy but a means of discovering your own and your partner's strength, balance, intuition, and mental stability. Instead of facing each other with distrust, fear, and competitiveness, you meet your practice partners with concentration, sincerity, and a sense of enjoyment.

•

Mitsugi Saotome

Crime studies have shown that most assaults occur between family members, estranged partners, by aggressors that are known to the victim. Anonymous attacks do occur, however, and in most cases the attacker chooses a person who looks like a victim. Walking confidently and carefully seems to discourage would-be attackers. It is ironic that the more one trains in this type of self-defense, the less likely one is called upon to use it on the street.

Martial artists rarely practice in a negative, frightened, or angry mind set. They feel that they are learning something fun, and that gives proven physical results, so they feel good. Although clearly the body is participating in the act of punching, kicking, grappling, or throwing, the spirit is not angry or unhappy. Quite the opposite kinds of energies are at work here in the *dojo*, as we have discussed in previous chapters.

Even while the intellect absorbs subtle nuances of technique, and knowledge of where exactly in the human body a counterattack will have the most effect, the brain remains clear of harmful intent. Students are admonished to focus their entire being on the flow of technique. They will defend themselves with maximum effort and yet in the visualization of the attack there is not an iota of hate. This is different from some of the more popular self-defense courses, in which participants are encouraged to use their fear and rage against attackers. Although some psychological therapists recommend such practice for those immobilized by fear or trauma from previous attacks, this technique is a distortion of the desired mind set of martial arts.

Martial artists are trained to expect the unexpected. Part of this is developing an alertness and preparedness that comes from being relaxed and comfortable with oneself. Attacks can happen in public spaces in broad daylight and also from sources one least expects. Self-defense against "bullies" might involve physical and mental attacks from strangers on the street, drivers in traffic, co-workers, school-mates, and even pushy people in the supermarket aisles. Rather than encouraging paranoia or abrasive attitudes, those involved in the martial arts seek to project a positive outlook that is helpful, confident, and capable. This allows them to respond in a manner appropriate to the perceived offense, rather than overreact, as often happens in such cases.

Teachers who stress only the sport aspect of the martial arts or insist that the only way to train is through combat-oriented, self-defense routines, are doing a disservice to their students. They are failing themselves and the general public by not sharing all that the martial arts can offer. They have abandoned the traditions and goals of the founders of these systems, who intended that the health and fitness benefits be available for everyone. The masters believed these benefits to be the most important aspect of their disciplines and that from good health, all else would follow.

Practicing martial arts is not like doing aerobics or playing tennis for an hour. It involves a change in your perspectives about your body, how you can develop and maintain your fitness and health, what you choose to do to take control of your life, and how your energy, spirit, and attitude will improve as a result of this different relationship. By engaging your mental and spiritual resources, a better equilibrium can be established. This progress can be gradual, like the small steps the martial artist takes to learn physical technique; but as the training proceeds,

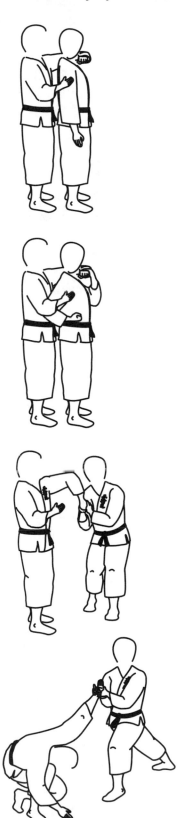

A defensive series of responses to an attack from behind, utilizing displacement and lowering of the center of gravity.

changes occur in the metabolism. This will produce alterations in the needs of the body, and therefore affect how the mind feels about it. Changes in desires and habits will result as well, making it easier to do things for oneself, such as eating well, that will help the body perform better. As training capabilities improve, the cycle continues, with mind, body, and spirit getting into "sync" and developing new patterns that improve health and happiness.

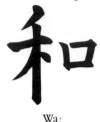

Wa:
harmony

Martial artists are usually thought of as highly disciplined, and most people think this is due to the strict regulations of the *dojo*. Although it is true that some schools are more militaristic than others, the purpose of such discipline is to ensure a safe training environment for everyone. By adhering to a code of behavior that places appropriate respect for the nature of the training and an environment conducive for learning, great strides can be taken. This is the framework of martial arts philosophy, within which the individual develops a self-restraint that results from enjoying the activity and seeing results.

The student still has to find the will to come to class, work hard, and be open to the teaching. By seeing progress in their personal lives, outside of the *dojo* as well as within, participants will make changes because they want to, not because they have to. These are the types of life-style changes that can be made permanent, because they work, because they are simple, and because they are acquired gradually. Most of us have experienced the failure of even the most well-intentioned lists of resolutions when we have set out to improve ourselves. Usually, the will is there, but we often attempt to make all the changes at once, and are miserable due to our lack of success.

The martial artist's interpretation of discipline does not require a rigid or unnatural imprisoning of emotion, desire, or experience. Rather, it is the bringing of these elements into balance with a well-rounded physical framework and an enlightened moderation that provides the practitioner with a truly personal defense. While one can take inspiration from a Zen monk and study long and hard to discover and illuminate the truth, it does not necessarily follow that one has to choose the ascetic life of the monk.

There are many influences in the modern world that we must fortify ourselves against. Pollution, overpopulation, urban decay, and natural disasters, all have stressful effects on our lives, but there seems to be little we can do about them. The "small steps" philosophy subscribes to the "think globally, act locally" approach to taking action. In the same way, martial artists defend against the smaller scale stresses of work-related problems or family demands by taking good care of themselves and helping those around them to do the same. Being able to avoid illness, injury, stress, and depression are skills far more likely to be actually needed than an ability to defeat an attacker in a dark alley, yet the same principles that the martial artist learns in the actual practice of personal defense can be used to fend off more mundane threats such as germs or tension. In the practice of *ippon kumite* (one-step sparring), for example, the student learns to analyze an attack and devise a strategy to meet it. He then practices it over and over in different variations so that it becomes second nature, effortless yet extremely effective.

The martial artist, when confronted with an opponent about to launch an attack, first tries to clearly identify the nature of the weapon: where is it (which hand or foot); where is it coming from; and the path of its trajectory (high, low, direct, or circular). Once those are ascertained, he will move out of the way of the assault. By ducking, sidestepping, moving backward, or even forward to get behind the attacker, his purpose is simply not to be there when the attack comes. As additional insurance—in case he reacted too slowly, or the attack was particularly strong and fast—he will deflect or if necessary block the blow. In so doing, he sets himself up for a counterattack, a way of fighting back that will neutralize the attack and control it so that it cannot be launched again. This calculated response can be thought of as a metaphor for the martial artist's approach to all aspects of personal defense.

The martial arts are not about going out and attacking what appears wrong in the world, nor about passively waiting for disaster to happen. Martial artists are engaged in studying how to control and utilize their bodies, thought processes, and emotions, in what appears to be self-defense against attack by others. However, the main purpose of acquiring these skills is to enable them to deal with other problems in their lives. More importantly, they want to just get on with the activity of living, not focusing on problems, but rather on solutions. Rather than as defense against potential armed attackers, the keen awareness of physical sensations, developed intellect, and the spiritual awakening that can result from the study of martial arts, is better put to use in the appreciation of a gentle sunrise, the cultivation of a garden, or as a volunteer in the community.

Wrist and Body Rotation Exercise
Front Stance

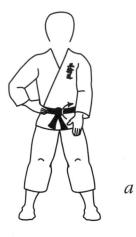

a

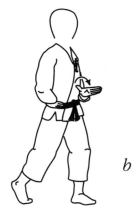

b

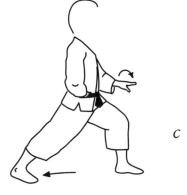

c

Stance: Begin in ready stance, facing front, feet shoulder width apart.

Action: Begin with the left wrist rotation, inside to outside, with the other hand resting on the hip. At the same time, pivot on the ball of the left foot, lifting the right heel. As the turn to the left and circle of hand is completed, place the right foot further backward and lower weight forward into front stance, *zenkutsu-dachi*. Be sure that the action is coordinated and smooth, without interruptions *(a, b & c)*. Exhale at the same time and repeat it ten times on each side.

As the second phase, add the other hand rotating from the elbow and finishing with a pushing down action with hands side by side *(d, e & f)*. Lead all the motion with the eyes first, followed by the head and then the hip.

This simple exercise can be applied as a defensive technique to break a crossing hold on the wrist with one or two hands.

The body rotation makes the wrist angle more effective for releasing the grip of the attacker, and the lowering of the center of gravity assists the downward force behind the partner's elbow joint.

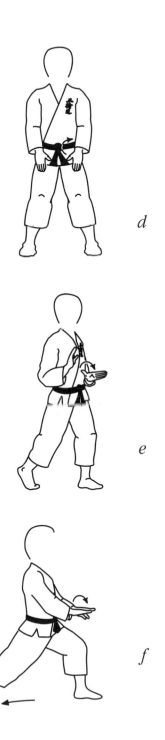

d

e

f

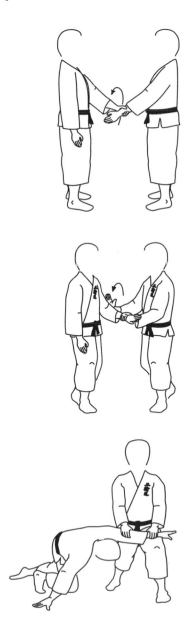

Two-Wrist Rotation

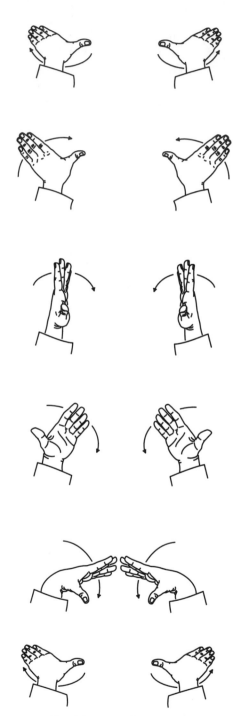

Stance: Can be done seated or standing but it is important to be able to breathe comfortably throughout.

Action: The rotation series is outside to inside, repeated ten times, and then inside to outside, ten circles as well. The exercise should be done slowly at first and then can be increased in speed. The exact hand position is important; it is not just a casual circling of the hands. Keep both elbows close to the body and train both sides equally. Focus on the exhalation phase of the breathing.

As an exercise, raise each knee alternately with the pulling motion. Exhale and *kiai* on the tenth repetition.

Outside-to-inside rotation

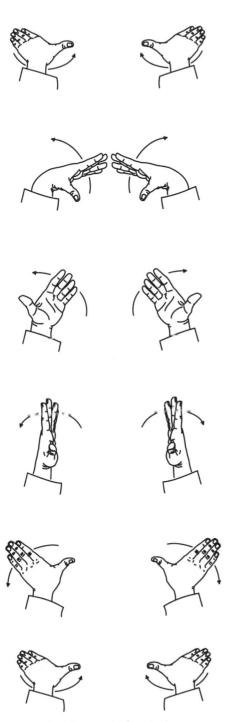

Inside-to-outside rotation

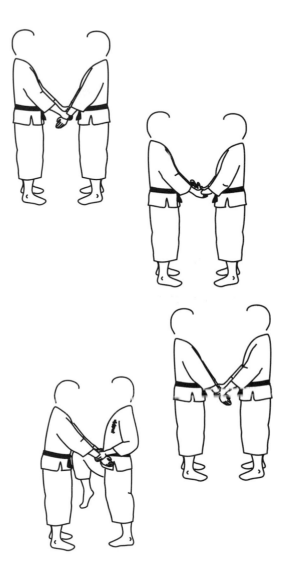

The application of the wrist rotation is a defensive maneuver that can also be practiced as an individual exercise. To defend against a double wrist grab, rotate the hand from the inside to outside position, grab the partner's wrists and pull toward your own hips, counterattacking with a knee to the front of your partner's body.

Gorindo Figure-Eight Exercise

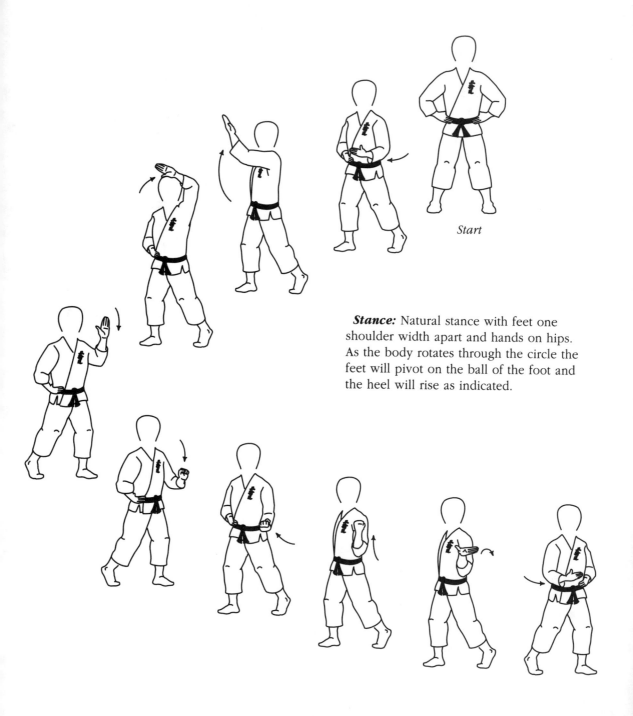

Start

Stance: Natural stance with feet one shoulder width apart and hands on hips. As the body rotates through the circle the feet will pivot on the ball of the foot and the heel will rise as indicated.

Action: Open the left hand into *shuto* (knife-hand) position, palms up. Keeping elbows in, move the hand across the body and up, pivoting the hips to the right. Inhale gently. As the hand passes back across above the head, palm out, pivot in the opposite direction. Imagine that you are describing a curved window frame. As the hand passes down the other side, led by the descending elbow, gently clench the hand into a fist, which is brought up the center line in an uppercut fashion as the body turns back again toward the right. The figure-eight cycle concludes with the hand opening into a tiger claw that rotates outward, slightly down, and pulls back as a finish. Empty the lungs completely. Ideally the full cycle should be completed in one long exhalation. Inhale during the transition of changing to the other hand and beginning in the other direction. Keep the body relaxed and loose in the hips, knees, and ankles, as you shift the weight from one leg to the other. Remember to raise heels in a natural turning. Repeat for a total of ten complete figure-eights.

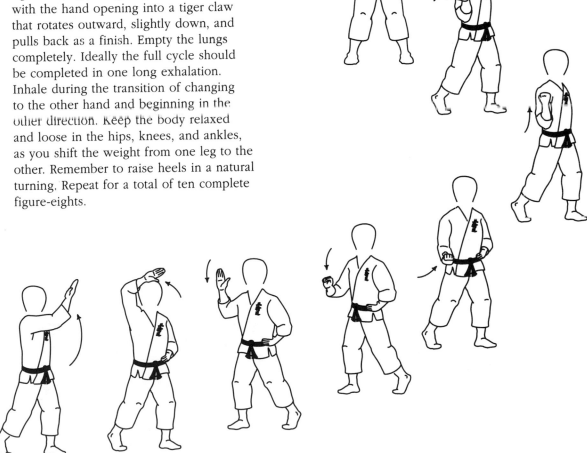

Examples of the application of the Figure-Eight Exercise in defensive situations.

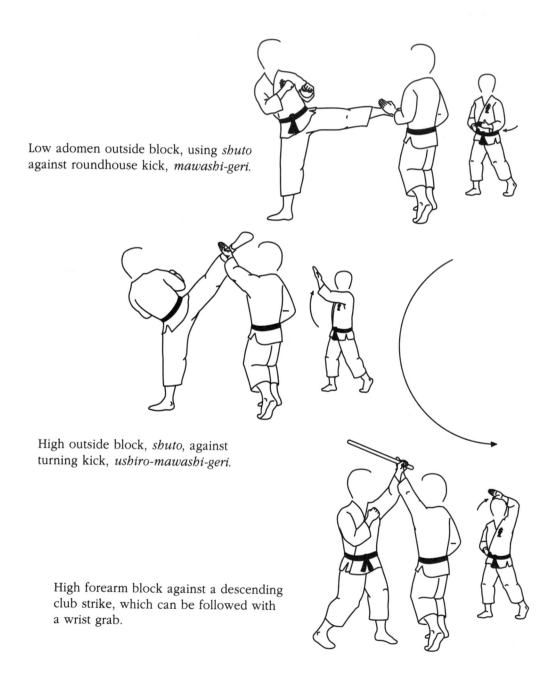

Low adomen outside block, using *shuto* against roundhouse kick, *mawashi-geri*.

High outside block, *shuto*, against turning kick, *ushiro-mawashi-geri*.

High forearm block against a descending club strike, which can be followed with a wrist grab.

Defense against a cross-wrist grab, with
outside wrist rotation and hip motion
that adds more pressure on the
partner's wrist joint.

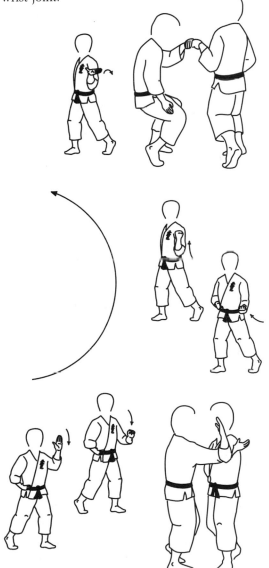

Trapping of the partner's arm
and application of pressure on
the elbow and shoulder joint
with a hip rotation and uppercut
motion.

Defense against a shoulder grab,
trapping partner's arm under the armpit.

Secrets of the Martial Arts

- Every man, woman, and child has the right to personal liberty, privacy, and autonomy. We adjust these rights within the reasonable limits imposed by our need to gather in social groups.

- Martial artists practice the art of self-defense in all its conventional aspects, but go further in using the same principles to avoid and deflect attacks on their physical, mental, and spiritual well-being.

- Strengthened spiritual fortitude and a well-developed sense of self allows us to deal with the emotions involved when misfortune does strike, and can be one of the most valuable benefits of martial arts training.

- It is precisely because of the respect, traditions, and attention to consistant progressive practice, that the long-term study of martial arts can offer a safe, effective approach to self-defense.

- Confidence and serenity come from having a healthy, strong body, trained reflexes, and experience in meeting an attack.

- Practicing a martial art involves a change in your perspectives about your body, how you can develop and maintain your fitness and health, what you choose to do to take control of your life, and how your energy, spirit, and attitude will improve as a result of this different relationship.

- The martial artist's interpretation of discipline does not require a rigid or unnatural imprisoning of emotion, desire or experience. Rather, it is the bringing of these elements into balance with a well-rounded physical framework and an enlightened moderation that provides the practitioner with a truly personal defense.

Chapter 9

Nurturing the Spirit

THERE is no way to comprehend quickly the total scope of the martial arts. There are many small and easy-to-take steps, good answers to sensible questions, and resounding *kiai* that complete a technique, but the whole picture doesn't fit into any one viewfinder. The many elements that make up the study of martial arts, and the interwoven layers of thought, action, and feelings that the practitioner brings to them, can be somewhat overwhelming. Students nevertheless usually find themselves on a path that brings order to their lives and enriches their daily experience. Although some participate just for the exercise, the philosophy is so deeply rooted in the practice that even those uninterested in it are still affected by it.

Martial artists, by virtue of their training, take part in a unique form of self-analysis. By confronting strengths and weaknesses on a direct physical level, students are constantly made aware of their mental and spiritual development. In this way, the body leads the mind on a path of discovery, even though the conscious ego may think the "self" is still in charge. This interplay is what keeps the sometimes arduous training fresh and interesting. Just keeping up with yourself is sufficiently engaging and exciting for one willing to proceed with an open mind, heart, and *hara*. There is no need to hide from companions along the way, let alone compete with them.

Nurturing the spirit is the key to unlocking any struggle between the body and the mind. Finding out what motivates you, gives you energy and joy, and sticking to the things you love can give meaning to your existence. These do not have to be grand schemes or accomplishments, but can be simple affirmations of personal choice and commitment.

The scent of a single blossom is enough to enrich the most dismal circumstances, if your character has been formed sufficiently to recognize its presence and allow its beauty passage. By following a personally chosen path through the confusion of modern life, a measure of peace can be obtained.

The study of a martial art is often likened to hiking a path up a mountain. It is an analogy common to spiritual undertakings as well, and recognizable to almost anyone who has embarked on a career, artistic endeavor, or any project that requires hard work over a long period of time.

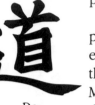

Do:
way

Further, the Way, *do*, is always one of "beginning again." The principle of *nyuanshin* can apply at every belt level, every class, every new technique. For martial artists in our modern systems, this idea must be carefully reinforced at the black-belt level. Most people think that only experts wear a black belt and that they are consequently not to be messed with. Very few realize that within most traditions, the black belt is only a beginning, and that there are upwards of nine or ten *dan* levels, or degrees, of black belt. From white belt to brown belt, the grade levels, are numbered in descending *kyu* (usually nine) with first *kyu* being the "rank" just before the transition to black belt, where the progression then ascends from *shodan, nidan* (first degree, second degree) and so on. The threshold the student must cross when accepting the responsibilities of the black belt is loaded with significance, especially in the West, where it is seen as a noteworthy accomplishment. The black-belt grading exam takes on harrowing proportions in some schools, and is a major event in the life of a *dojo*. Even though the schools may be part of large associations and may have boards of examiners and written requirements for the black-belt level and test, tradition still holds that the black belt represents the transmission of knowledge, trust, and responsibility from teacher to student. The value of the black belt and its meaning to others is directly related to who conveyed it. It is a recognition that they felt the student was prepared to move on to another level of learning and comprehension in the martial arts. The aspect of that tradition that is less well known is the reciprocal acknowledgment on the part of the student of an even more stringent code of respect and duty, and an obligation to uphold the virtues and teaching standards of the teacher and the school.

Although there is usually great honor accorded the newly minted (and exhausted) *yudansha* (black-belt holders) on the night of their exam, the next day that they walk into the *dojo* to train, they are traditionally treated no differently than new white belts. Often the *sensei* will even be more strict and relentless in the pursuit of their errors

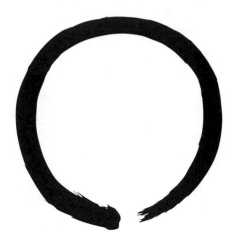

*As in the visual arts, the
martial arts seek to
express the inner state
of mind and spirit.*

and weaknesses. In some schools, where the wearing of the *hakama* is traditional for black-belt level, *yudansha* find themselves suddenly asked to perform in this long flowing "skirt" that trips up the feet and binds legs, until they become accustomed to moving in it. It is thought that this is a not so subtle joke played upon them to ensure that their *hara* does not swell, and they are reminded of their "beginning again" status in the *dojo*.

In some schools a black belt is automatically referred to as *sensei*, acknowledging the senior rank and distinction of one who has traveled the path before. *Sempai* is the term by which junior students refer to their seniors, although in martial arts the term has come to mean assistant to the teacher. In some schools these terms are designations given only to particular students who have been recognized for exceptional ability and teaching responsibilities. In other traditions it would be unheard of for someone below third or fourth *dan* to be referred to as *sensei*.

Likewise the title of master (whether *renshi*, *shihan*, or *kyoshi*), has different meanings in different schools. The primary teacher at a school, if his knowledge, experience, and *dan* ranking are appropriate, may certainly be thought of as a master, but that respect may in some cases only be accorded to the head of a *ryu*, someone older, of higher rank and either the founder or the designated heir of the school's traditions.

There is no standardization of *dan* ranking, and designations of *sensei* or master titles, nor could there be, given the numerous schools, *ryu*, styles, lines, and offshoots that exist. There are many excellent teachers who teach independently of any association that might convey advanced ranking upon them, just as there are, unfortunately, instructors of high rank who have been conferred titles for political reasons and are not necessarily more skilled or better teachers.

This situation makes it difficult for newcomers to the martial arts to choose a school and style of training that is appropriate for them. It is another situation in which *caveat emptor* applies, and prospective students should ask for recommendations, visit many schools, and observe classes carefully before signing up. There are many questions that beginners might pose to teachers of prospective schools, but remember that they are just as concerned about the attitude, motivations, and background of potential students. If you are truly looking for a teacher to guide you on a Way in the martial arts, don't expect to be catered to like a customer.

The credentials and experience of teachers is important in assessing their program. Their attitude toward themselves, their students, and their school will be reflected in their personal views and deportment, how they relate to their students, and the concern they show for the health and safety of the students in their care. The cleanliness and good repair of the *dojo* and equipment, the length of warm-up and cool-down exercises, and quality of the assistant instructors and senior students are all important indicators that can be observed and assessed. If you wish to be accepted at a good school it is important that you conduct your search and investigations with respect, care, and an open mind. No good teacher would be displeased that you returned to his school after visiting others, but don't be offended if you also are examined before being admitted. Traditionally, an eager student was rejected several times, and had to show his desire and perseverance by camping on the doorstep or sweeping the grounds for many weeks before being allowed in the door.

Natural Associations

OBSERVATIONS and imagination reveal associations between natural elements and qualities sought by the martial artist.

WATER	EARTH	TREE	AIR
fluid	rock	growth & change	breath
hard, soft	ancient	pliant	fire
changes form	solid	sturdy	free
essential	shape	grace	disperse
waves	soothe	longevity	concentrate
calm	soft	strength	flow
current	cool	reach	inspiration
refresh	metamorphic	transformation	sing
float		form	wind
vessel			

Dojo Layout

"The dojo is vertical in experience and horizontal in co-operation."

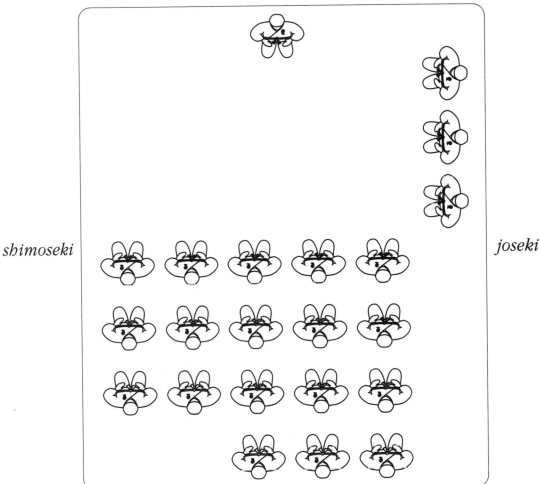

shomen

shimoseki

joseki

shimoza

SHOMEN: upper seating area, reserved for *sensei*, teachers or honored guests.

Joseki: upper-right side, where the *yudansha* (black-belt practitioners) sit.

Shimoseki: lower-left side, area with seating for visitor or spectators, at the left of the upper seat or *shomen*.

Shimoza: lower seating area, usually where the additional equipment for training is stored.

When lining up for class, the highest-level students will be to the right front of the *shomen* area. Students form rows across and behind in descending order of belt level. If more than one student is of the same belt level, then the one with the longest time in that grade will be to the right. If both have the same time training, priority is given to the one who started earliest. If they have the same starting date, then the eldest will line up to the right.

Visitors to the *dojo* go to the rear of the class unless invited to do otherwise by the *sensei*.

The probationary period does not end when you pay your fees or begin classes. The doors swing both ways in most *dojo*, and sometimes it takes a while to find the right fit of teacher and student, learning environment, and peer group. Again, the practitioner and school must exercise a balance between loyalty and compatibility. It is important for the student to recognize that there will be moments of doubt and discouragement along the Way; overcoming these is part of the training. Many times the rewards are reaped after a period of discontentment that has been resolved by practice, practice, practice. Understanding comes upon reaching higher ground, from which things appear clearer.

The beginner's mind is an attitude that one must possess before a committed and productive study of the martial arts is possible. Yet Western society does not always prepare us for this approach to serious learning. We do not have the traditional respect for the teacher that is inculcated by Eastern cultures and philosophies. By demanding from our leaders instant success at the lowest possible cost in time and effort we have a tendency to get what we pay for.

Martial arts offer a unique opportunity to those wishing to engage themselves fully. For both teachers and students the ancient traditions and knowledge offer a way to focus their energies in the company of others who are like-minded. The immediacy of the learning process, its rigid boundaries, and precise demands actually free practitioners in many ways. By not having to re-invent the wheel, decode and plan, compromise and politicize, they can simply come to the *dojo* and "do." The exercise program is there waiting, with partners eager to practice and a teacher willing to help sort things out, plus the collective wisdom of centuries to ponder and enrich the spirit. By accepting a chosen path you will benefit from not only your own experiences, but those of your fellow students, your teacher, her teacher, and the others who have gone before. There is such a great deal to learn that a basic road map makes it more enjoyable. It is no small thing that advanced students, regardless of the Way they have followed, find that the important lessons at the root of their various Ways have proved to be the same. Such paths have a habit of converging as they approach the summit. This is where much of the sharing of knowledge and traditions has occurred in the martial arts. It is almost as if the proverbial *yogi* on the mountain leave their lonely caves at night, and get together for a good time around the campfire, sharing stories and songs after the tourists have gone home.

Beginning in the training of one's body, practice continues with the training of one's spirit. Finally one realizes that body and spirit are not two things but one. This is true practice.

•

Shigeru Egami
1912–80

The camaraderie of shared experience in the *dojo* is one of the most rewarding features of martial Ways. It is the fellowship of individuals who understand something of each other's journey. Even when guided by the same teacher, two paths are never identical; the internal work and the difficulties overcome shape the process into unique experiences. A martial artist is not afraid to walk alone.

The study of martial arts is a complete package. However, it offers many things to different people and, like most activities, what students receive depends on what they bring of themselves to the table. The spirit of the martial arts always demands going back to basics and polishing the diamond. Like a meridian of *ki* energy, the martial spirit can be accessed in many ways and from different directions. The teachings can be called upon to inspire and enable the integration of mind and body, to reach beyond an uncomfortable rut and find a smooth groove. The practice of martial arts will improve the health and fitness of the whole being; it gives individuals the fortitude to let go of patterns that are no longer serving them well, and provides the strength and will to knock down what is known to be less than satisfactory and to build again on a firmer foundation.

Rebirth and creativity are central to a spiritual understanding of martial arts, but one can approach them without being religious or esoteric. By staying rooted in the physical, students get to observe practical examples every time they train. Their experience is very tactile, real, and in the moment, and from it can be distilled the motivation for pursuing health and fitness as a lifestyle, not just as a leisure time activity or a medical prescription.

Martial arts teaches students to strike exactly where they want, not just where they can. This attitude and ability changes everything about what is possible in their lives. It empowers individuals to achieve goals, but also to enjoy the process of getting there. The simple secret of martial arts training is to "breathe, relax, and smile." These are the warrior's shield against adversity.

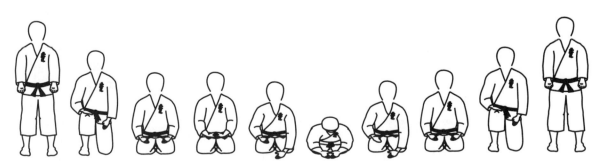

Assuming seiza *position followed by the bow,* zarei.

This secret weapon is cultivated in the practice of *zazen* breathing and meditation. Although we know that this is usually practiced in *seiza*, seated meditation, martial artists also seek to utilize this mind state and breathing regimen in full motion. Knowing that one's central core, both physical and mental, can be protected and revitalized by breathing and remaining calm allows the spirit to be more courageous, adventurous, and generous. This nurturing of spirit circles back to make the body and mental processes stronger.

The mind state that one is trying to achieve in *zazen* and eventually to access in all aspects of the training is referred to as *hishiryo*, or "no mind." Like many of the concepts that come from Zen into the martial arts, the idea is simple but the explanation complicated. The understanding of it is intuitive and comes from practice, not deductive reasoning. "No mind" is a state of being that is free of conscious thought yet very aware and essential. In action it is all action, at rest it is pure rest. This state is not something that one can pursue, for it flees from any attempt to capture or control it. For most students it can be glimpsed only momentarily, but that instant of *satori*, Zen enlightenment, in which one is connected to the universe, can be tantalizing and encourages renewed effort to repeat and extend the experience.

Zazen practice helps the body, mind, and spirit come into an intimate awareness and harmony that in turn allows for this emptying of the mind. The ego must be met and undressed. Thoughts and distractions cannot be avoided, but like each breath, they are encouraged to pass on as they came, unaffected and undiminished. Beginners find it difficult to let go of their conscious apprehension and understanding of the external world. Other methods of meditation use *mantras*, repetitive sayings or sounds, to focus the mind in one direction away from intruding thoughts, but in *zazen* this initial exercise takes the form of concentrating on the breathing pattern and the flow of energy though the body.

One common traditional metaphor for *zazen* and *hishiryo* is that of the mind as the reflection of the moon upon the water. Although wind, waves, and currents may act upon the surface of the water and diffract the image, there is still light being reflected, the moon still exists, the

To renew applies when we are fighting with the enemy, and an entangled spirit arises where there is no possible resolution. We must abandon our efforts, think of the situation in a fresh spirit then win in the new rhythm. To renew, when we are deadlocked with the enemy, means that without changing circumstances we change our spirit and win through a different technique.

•

Miyamoto Musashi
1584–1645

water exists, and when calm returns, the image again becomes clear and untroubled.

We have discussed how controlled abdominal breathing and correct spinal alignment can produce a physiological state that supports the flow of energy and relaxes the mind. The martial arts practitioner learns as well that these promote the nurturing of *shen*, the spirit-mind. This integration of mental and spiritual resources is what martial arts training seeks to achieve.

Students attempt to identify and connect with this energy in all aspects of their practice, and the more they are able to do this, the easier technique becomes. As training progresses, the connection occurs more often, and eventually students understand that this union, this *kiai*, is the true objective. *Kihon, kata, kumite* and even *zazen* sitting are all in aid of flow, balance, and serenity, goals of the simple directive to breathe, relax, and smile.

It is in this way that martial artists can bring full commitment of body, mind, and spirit to the moment that they are in, the here and now. Their goal becomes expanding or stretching that moment until it flows directly into the next, seamlessly and without hesitation. The martial arts master, in action, is able to project his intention into the next moment with such energy that the body is pulled into that space as if sucked into a vacuum. He is seeking to extend his being as a series of points into a line, by fully forming each breath, each intention, and each transformation of energy.

This then, is the "secret" of the martial arts. Everyone who comes to the training has the opportunity to access such potential even as a beginner. Many people start to train because they have had similar experiences in sports, arts, or intellectual studies, and found out that the

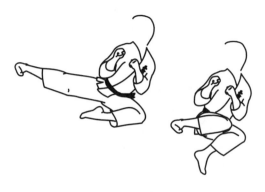
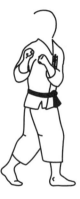
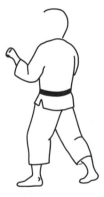

Kicking with kiai, *the dynamic expression of spirit in technique.*

martial arts *dojo* was a place to seriously study this phenomena. Others are just lucky to discover the possibilties along the way. What separates the master from the beginner is practice, practice, practice, and the ability to integrate its results into their lives.

The master also has the ability to teach this knowledge to others. It is not enough to arrive at this level of understanding and keep it to himself. Not only is this selfish and disrespectful of the traditions of the martial arts, it means that the practitioner is not allowing his knowledge and ability to be examined, reevaluated, and refreshed. A true master is still a student and opens his mind and *hara* to new experiences and ways of looking at things.

This is also the way in which the martial arts, as a whole, continues to prosper. The students of today owe it to their seniors to share what they have learned from them, and pass it on undiluted and respectful of the traditions. They also have a responsibility to examine the teachings and their own practice with due diligence, looking beneath the surface for meaning and understanding. New information and alternative approaches should be welcomed and allowed to influence the training if they help to illuminate or reinforce the essential principles of the martial arts, but caution must be exercised. When a good understanding of a traditional path has been reached, one is in a better position to evaluate its usefulness and a future course of action. Some new paths lead to dead ends, and others have a tendency to circle around and find their way back to roads already taken.

Martial arts provide a philosophy for living well. The basic ideas, methods, and systems for learning and teaching them have been honed and improved for many years, across centuries and cultural borders. The training provides aesthetic and intellectual influences that inform and engage the individual in an integrated balance of body and mind. Health and fitness of the body and spirit are at the heart of the martial arts, and its methods for improving character and developing a moderate discipline are what make it so effective and rewarding. The benefits include a stronger body, a more flexible outlook, and an enhanced ability to focus on the priorities of a positive existence.

The study of martial arts has changed many lives. It can have a profound influence on the way one sees, thinks, feels, and moves. By providing a framework for mental and physical awareness and evaluation, individuals can actively take charge of their health and happiness. It is a path of simple steps and deep satisfaction.

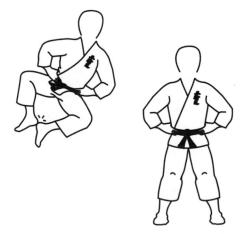

Further Readings

- The authors suggest these titles for those beginning on the path.

Akishige, Yoshiharu. *Psychological studies on zen.* Tokyo: Zen Institute of Kumazawa University, 1970.

Choi, Hong Hi. *Tae kwon do, the Korean art of self-defence* (15 volumes). Mississauga, ON: International Taekwon-do Federation, 1993.

Chun, Richard. *Advancing in tae kwon do.* New York: Harper & Row, Publishers, Inc., 1982.

Chun, Richard. *Tae kwon do, the Korean martial art.* New York: Harper & Row, Publishers, Inc., 1976.

Davey, H. E. *Unlocking the secrets of aiki-jujutsu.* Indianapolis: Masters Press, 1997.

- Deshimaru, Taisen. *The zen way to the martial arts.* 1982. New York: Penguin Books, Inc., 1991.

Draeger, Donn F. *Classical budo.* New York: Weatherhill, Inc., 1973.

Draeger, Donn F. *Classical bujutsu.* New York: Weatherhill, Inc., 1973.

- Draeger, Donn F. *Modern bujutsu and budo.* New York: Weatherhill, Inc., 1974.

- Egami, Shigeru. *The heart of karate-do.* Tokyo: Kodansha International, Ltd., 1976.

Feldenkrais, Moshe. *Body and mature behaviour.* New York: International Universities Press, Inc.,1979.

Funakoshi, Gichin. *Karate-do kyohan, the master text* (translated by Tsutomu Oshima). Tokyo: Kodansha International, Ltd., 1973.

Funakoshi, Gichin. *Karate-do nyumon, the master introductory text* (translated by John Teramoto). Tokyo: Kodansha International, Ltd., 1988.

- Funakoshi, Gichin. *Karate-do, my way of life.* Tokyo: Kodansha International, Ltd., 1975.

Gleason, William. *The spiritual foundations of aikido.* Rochester, VT: Destiny Books, 1995.

- Gluck, Jay. *Zen combat.* 1962. Revised and enlarged edition. Ashiya, Japan: Personally Oriented, 1996.

Guyton, Arthur C., M.D. *Textbook of medical physiology.* Philadelphia: W. B. Saunders Company, 1986.

Harrison, Ernest J. *The fighting spirit of Japan.* 1955. Woodstock, NY: The Overlook Press, 1982.

Hashimoto, Keizo, M.D. *Sotai, natural exercise* (translated by Herman Aihara). 1977. Oroville, CA: George Ohsawa Macrobiotic Foundation, 1981.

Hashimoto, Keizo, M.D. with Kawakami, Yoshiaki. *Sotai, balance and health through natural movement* (translated by Stephen Brown and Richard Held). Tokyo: Japan Publications, Inc., 1983.

Hirai, Tomio, M.D. *Zen meditation and psychotherapy.* Tokyo: Japan Publications, Inc., 1989.

Huard, Pierre Alphonse, and Wong, Ming. *Oriental methods of mental and physical fitness* (translated by Donald N. Smith). 1971. New York: Funk & Wagnalls Publishing Co., Inc., 1977.

• Hyams, Joe. *Zen in the martial arts.* 1979. New York: Bantam Books, 1982.

• Iedwab, Claudio, and Standefer, Roxanne. *Gorindo: standard manual.* Bancroft, ON: Sensei Uensei Books, 1997.

Journal of Asian Martial Arts. Erie, PA: Via Media Publishing, Co.

Kano, Jigoro. *Kodokan judo.* 1955. Revised edition. Tokyo: Kodansha International, Ltd., 1980.

Kauz, Herman P. *A path to liberation: a spiritual and philosophical approach to the martial arts.* Woodstock, NY: The Overlook Press, 1992.

• Kauz, Herman P. *The martial spirit.* Woodstock, NY: The Overlook Press, 1977.

Kim, Richard. *The classical man.* Hamilton, ON: Masters Publication, 1982.

Kim, Richard. *The weaponless warriors.* Burbank, CA: Ohara Publications, Inc., 1974.

Koizumi, Gunji. *My study of judo.* New York: Sterling Publications Co., Inc. 1960.

Lam Kam Chuen. *The way of energy: mastering the Chinese art of internal strength with chi kung exericise.* New York: Simon & Schuster, Inc., 1991.

Lee, Bruce. *Tao of jeet kune do.* 1975. Santa Clarita, CA: Ohara Publications, Inc., 1991.

Lee, Bruce. *The Tao of gung fu* (The Bruce Lee Library, vol. 2, edited by John Little). Boston: Tuttle Publishing, 1997.

Liao, Waysun. *T'ai chi classics.* Boston: Shambala, 1977.

Lowry, Dave. *Sword and brush: the spirit of the martial arts.* Boston: Shambala Publications, 1995.

Mann, Felix, M.B. *Acupunture: the ancient Chinese art of healing and how it works scientifically.* 1962. Revised edition. New York: Random House, Inc., 1972.

McCarthy, Patrick. *The bible of karate, Bubishi.* Rutland: Charles E. Tuttle Company, Inc., 1995.

Mifune, Kyuzo. *Canon of judo* (translated by K. Sugai). Tokyo: Seibundo-Shinkosha Publishing Co. Ltd., 1960.

Morizawa, Jackson S. *The secret of the target.* 1984. New York: Routledge & Kegan Paul, Inc., 1988.

Musashi, Miyamoto. *A book of five rings* (translated by Victor Harris). Woodstock, NY: The Overlook Press, 1974.

Nakamura, Takashi. *Oriental breathing therapy*. Tokyo: Japan Publications, Inc., 1981.

Oyama, Matsutatsu. *Advanced karate*. Tokyo: Japan Publications, Inc., 1970.

Oyama, Matsutatsu. *The kyokushin way*. Tokyo: Japan Publications, Inc., 1979.

Oyama, Matsutatsu. *This is karate* (translated by Richard L Gage).1973. Revised edition. Tokyo: Japan Publications, Inc., 1980.

Payne, Peter. *Martial arts, the spiritual dimension*. New York: the Crossroad Publishing Company, 1981.

Reed, William. *Ki: a road that anyone can walk*. Tokyo: Japan Publications, Inc., 1992.

• Salzman, Mark. *Iron and silk*. New York: Random House, Inc., 1987.

Saotome, Mitsugi. *Aikido and the harmony of nature*. 1986. Boston: Shambala Publications, 1993.

Sekida, Katsuki. *Zen training*. New York: Weatherhill, Inc., 1975.

Soho, Takuan. *The unfettered mind* (translated by William Scott Wilson). Tokyo: Kodansha International, Ltd., 1986.

Stevens, John. *The secrets of aikido*. Boston: Shambala Publications, 1995.

Stux, Gabriel, and Pomeranz, Bruce. *Basics of acupunture*. Berlin: Springer-Verlag, 1988.

• Suzuki, Shunryu. *Zen mind, beginner's mind*. New York: Weatherhill, Inc., 1970.

• Tohei, Koichi. *Book of ki: a co-ordinating mind and body in daily life*. Tokyo: Japan Publications, Inc., 1979.

• Tohei, Koichi. *Ki in daily life*. Tokyo: Japan Publications, Inc., 1978.

• Ueshiba, Morihei. *Budo. teaching of the founder of aikido* (translated by John Stevens). Tokyo: Kodansha International, Ltd., 1991.

Wile, Douglas. *Lost T'ai-chi classics from the late Ch'ing dynasty*. Albany, NY: State University of New York Press, Inc., 1996.

Yagyu, Munenori. *The sword and the mind* (translated by Hiroaki Sato). Woodstock, NY: The Overlook Press, 1986.

Yuasa, Yasuo. *The body, self-cultivation, and ki-energy* (translated by Shigenori Nagatomo and Monte S. Hull). Albany, NY: State University of New York Press, Inc., 1993.

Contact the Authors

For more information about Gorindo, "the Friendly Martial Art" and other publications, programs, and research of the authors of this book, please visit us at our website: www.gorindo.com or e-mail: gorindo@hotmail.com or by real mail: P.O. Box 1961, Bancroft, ON, Canada, K0L 1C0.

The "weathermark" identifies this book as a production of Weatherhill, Inc., publishers of fine books on Asia and the Pacific. Editorial supervision: Ray Furse. Design and page composition: Claudio Iedwab and Roxanne Standefer. Illustration: Claudio Iedwab. Cover photo: Roxanne Standefer. Production supervision: Bill Rose. Pre-press output: Lazerline. Printing and binding: R. R. Donnelley. The typeface used is Garamond.